THE EASIEST DIETS EVER

Instant Weight Loss!

Doctor Approved!

Lose *10* pounds in *10* days – & Keep It Off!

By Bill Nagler, M.D.

American Media, Inc.

INSTANT WEIGHT LOSS
Lose 10 pounds in 10 days & keep it off!

Copyright © 2004 AMI Books, Inc.
Cover design: Carlos Plaza
Interior design: Debbie Browning

ISBN: 1-932270-40-x

First printing: June 2004
Printed in the United States of America

10 9 8 7 6 5 4 3 2 1

Table Of Contents

Implosion Therapy For Weight Loss
Making Implosion Therapy Work For You

Introduction:
Doctor's Note

I've been in the trenches fighting fat for 20 years. During that time, I've treated more than 10,000 patients. Chances are, if you happened to live in the Detroit area any time during the past two decades and you saw a diet doctor, you saw me. From my experience, there is no magic bullet, potion or pill that will miraculously burn fat and keep it off forever. There is no man behind the curtain. The emperor is naked. It is unlikely that you have in your hands the perfect life-changing diet that will make you slim forever.

What this book offers you is a way to lose a bucket of weight in a hurry. You'll also be able to keep it off, too — at least until the reunion or cruise or anniversary or whatever. But soon after your landmark event, if you're like most people, you'll put back on every ounce. But don't worry. When you're ready to get back on the diet wagon, you can take it off again.

My Crash Diets are not forever, but for

quick weight loss right now. You can lose a quick 30 pounds for your high school reunion that's two months away. Or you can shed that unwanted 20 pounds in time for your anniversary in less than five weeks. Or you can to take off that last stubborn five pounds to look your best this Saturday night.

This is not the last diet you're ever going to go on, or the second to last. My diet is not meant to change your eating habits forever or make you model-slim for eternity. I may give you the jump-start you need to lose weight (and keep it off) over the long haul, but we will talk more about that later.

Bottom line, you can expect my Crash Diets to help you lose a bunch of weight in a hurry. You can lose five to 10 pounds this week and drop about five pounds every week thereafter.

When you do reach your goal, don't despair. Despite my doomsday feelings, you can keep your weight off a bit longer with my maintenance program. If you follow my No-Brainer Maintenance Program (See Section 3), you can double the time you stay thin. It is so easy, no one will know that you are on maintenance unless you tell them. But forget about that for now. We'll talk about maintenance after the reunion, anniversary or Saturday night date.

The diet programs outlined in this book are all very low-calorie diets. So, please consult your doctor before going on my 10-Days-10-Pounds-Off Program (See page 78), my 500 Diet (See page 93) or any of the programs in this book. See your personal physician first. Remove one of the diet tear-out sheets in this book and give it to your doctor at the time of your visit. Get medical approval before starting any weight-loss program. See Appendix I for the tear-out sheets for my diets. If your doctor doesn't want you to go on my diets, don't.

SECTION 1

The Virtue Of Weight Cycling

There are many factors that contribute to weight gain. The most common is eating too much. Medical causes of obesity are rare, but include inherited genetic characteristics; glandular disorders of the thyroid, pituitary, adrenal and sex glands, and metabolic disorders such as diabetes or hypoglycemia. Certain medications, such as cortisone, certain antidepressants and birth control pills, can contribute to weight gain. Psychological factors may also play a role.

Regardless of the cause, obesity can be treated. Obesity is a problem that must be treated and controlled. The reason is simple. Weighing too much increases your risk for developing many health problems. You can lower your health risks by losing as little as 10 to 20 pounds,[1] whether now or again and again. Some of these health problems include:

- Type-2 diabetes
- Heart disease and stroke
- Cancer
- Sleep apnea

- Osteoarthritis
- Gallbladder disease
- Fatty liver disease

Taking weight off and putting it back on again is not a bad thing. It's called weight cycling and, despite what popular media has said, weight cycling or yo-yo dieting is actually good for you. More precisely, weight cycling is far better for you than staying fat. In a study published in the *International Journal of Obesity*, Italian researchers concluded that there are no adverse cardiovascular effects associated with repeated weight loss and gain. They also found that weight cycling didn't affect body composition and body fat distribution.[2]

So, you're down 30 pounds. You stay there for a while, then during the next six months you put every ounce back on. You're actually healthier having lost weight and put it back on, than not having lost weight at all.

Extra weight adds stress to your heart. Every pound of fat requires your heart to pump a mile of blood a day. So, if you are down 30 pounds, that is 30 miles of blood that your heart no longer has to pump. Not only that, blood tends to be denser when you are overweight. Dense blood has more cholesterol and fatty acids in it, stressing the heart, elevating your blood pressure. Even when you gain back five, 10 or 15 pounds, your heart is still not working as hard as it would if you had maintained your weight of 160. Losing weight took stress off of your heart, at least for a while. Losing weight, even temporarily, reduces your risk of heart disease, stroke and cancer as well as relieves stress to the bones and joints, which can decrease symptoms of back pain and arthritis.

My program is designed to drop a bucket of weight in a hurry. You're probably going to put it all back on again. While your weight is down, you're slimmer and healthier. If you are committed, disciplined and following maintenance, there is a chance you can maintain your weight loss. But more about maintenance later.

The Virtue Of Crash Diets

My diets are not meant for long-term weight loss, but for a quick fix. However, according to Swedish researchers, very low-calorie diets, like mine, can be efficient for long-term weight loss. Lantz et al. reported in the *Journal of Internal Medicine* that the combination of an initial diet low in calories with behavior modification and an active follow-up period may be an efficient therapeutic approach.[3] Following 96 Swedish Obese Study subjects for eight years, the scientists found that those on very low-calorie diets maintained a three- to 10-pound weight loss. They concluded that those subjects who *completed* the program maintained a greater amount of weight loss than those who did not.

You know from experience that when you lose weight, it is very likely that you're going to gain every ounce back. And you probably think that is a very bad thing. I disagree.

The fact that you can lose weight is a good thing. If you can do it once, you can do it two or three times. Unless you want to radically change your lifestyle, the only way you can keep weight off is to go on and off diets. Just make sure that the diets are safe, protein sufficient and effective. My diets are all of these things. You can lose weight on my crash diets, keep it off for a while, and then go back and lose the weight again. And again and again.

To keep your weight off as long as possible, follow my No-Brainer Maintenance (See Section 3). Chances are that being human and not exercising, your weight will gradually creep back on again. But No-Brainer Maintenance can double the time you stay thin, based on the experience of thousands of my patients.

How Long Can You
Be On A Crash Diet?

Most of my patients stay on my programs anywhere from three days (to drop a quick five pounds) to three to four weeks (to drop a quick 15-20 pounds). In general, I don't recommend crash dieting for much more than one to two months at a time, even under medical supervision. Dieting is hard, hard work, and you need to give yourself a break. Take a week or two off after a month of dieting if you still have weight you want to lose and follow No-Brainer Maintenance. After a couple of weeks on No-Brainer, go back to my 10-Days-10-Pounds-Off Program, Dr. Nagler's 500 Diet or any of my other crash diet programs.

Assume that you want to drop a quick 10-40 pounds and you have your personal physician's approval. The best way to start is to jump in with both feet. Follow either my 10-Days-10-Pounds-Off Program or Dr. Nagler's 500 Diet, outlined in Section 2. Follow either program from three days (to drop a quick five) to one to two months (to drop 20-40 pounds).

Ketosis: The Fat-Burning State

Ketogenic Diets are very low carbohydrate diets. Ketosis is the process of dissolving fat and breaking it down into ketones, which are released through the breath and the urine. In ketosis, you are using fat for body fuel instead of sugar. The way to get into ketosis is to eat protein and to eliminate carbohydrates (starches and sweets) from your diet.

Using sugar or carbohydrates for fuel elevates your insulin level. Insulin converts excess carbohydrates into fat. If you have a tendency to eat too many carbohydrates, guess what can happen? You can store more fat, which can make you gain weight.

As you decrease carbohydrates in your diet, your insulin level drops. On a low-carbohydrate or ketogenic diet, insulin levels are low enough so that fat is burned and not stored. To be in ketosis, most people's carbohydrate intake needs to be between 10 and 20 grams a day. There are carbohydrate-counter books available that give you the exact number of carbohydrates contained in most foods.

In general, lean meat, chicken, fish and

some cheeses have zero carbohydrates. Grains, either whole or processed, have a very high carbohydrate count. Vegetables vary in their carbohydrate count. Sweet vegetables such as carrots and corn have a high carbohydrate count while watery, leafy vegetables like lettuce and spinach have low amounts of carbohydrates. Most fruits contain a lot of carbohydrates. Some fruits are worse than others. For example, grapes are high and strawberries are low.

The more grams of carbohydrates your body takes in, the slower your weight loss. If you're not careful and your carbohydrates go much above 20 grams per day, most people go out of ketosis and are not in an efficient fat-burning state. My 10-Days-10-Pounds-Off Program and 500 Diets make dieting simpler and weight loss quicker by cutting out foods that are high in carbohydrates. Counting carbohydrates is not necessary. Your food choices are simple and straight-forward.

The weight loss from a ketogenic diet is primarily fat tissue stored in the abdomen, waist, hips and thighs. Non-ketogenic diets, on the other hand, tend to be protein deficient and can result in a loss of normal essential muscle tissue. Muscle loss tends to create a pale, shallow appearance of the face and neck, and can produce symptoms of malnutrition such as hunger, fatigue, dizziness, lightheadedness, dehydration, lethargy, irritability and mild depression. Dieters on non-ketogenic diets often complain of losing weight from the wrong areas, too.

Being on a ketogenic diet gives you a metabolic advantage. Studies have shown that calorie-for-calorie, you will lose weight faster on a ketogenic diet than on any other type of weight-loss program.

Checking For Ketosis

To make sure you are in a fat-burning state, you must check your urine daily for ketosis. The best way to do this is with Ketostix (available at any drugstore). Make sure to buy Ketostix that test for urine ketones. Also check the expiration date of your Ketostix before using them. Dip the colored end of a Ketostix strip into a fresh urine specimen or pass it through a stream of urine. After 15 seconds compare the color of your strip with the color chart on the side of your Ketostix bottle.

If your strip is medium pink, you are in small or moderate ketosis, which is where you want to be. If the strip shows pale pink or beige, you are not in ketosis. If this is the case, you need to eliminate more carbohydrates from your diet. If the strip shows medium or dark purple, you are dehydrated and must drink more water.

Metabolic Setpoint: Your Fat-Regulating System

A ketogenic diet can also help to lower Metabolic Setpoint. Metabolic setpoint is the weight your body is genetically programmed to weigh. According to Robert Pool in his book *Fat: Fighting the Obesity Epidemic*, your level of body fatness, just like your body temperature and blood sugar, is kept within a tight range. Any attempt to fall below or rise above that setpoint significantly can be met with resistance.

Let's say you weigh 160 pounds and you diet your way down to 130 pounds. Although you are 30 pounds lighter than when you started your diet, you still experience the hunger you had at 160 pounds. So any time your willpower fades, or someone gives you a dirty look, or you are stressed, you eat and eat, until you eventually get back up to 160 pounds. The reason that you regained weight is that 160 pounds is your setpoint. Your setpoint is genetically predetermined. It is the amount of weight that your body is physiologically programmed to weigh.

Look at your parents and siblings. You likely have a similar build to at least one of your family members. Most people in the same family are shaped the same way. They all carry about the same weight for their height and bone-structure. This is your genetically determined setpoint. Your setpoint controls how hungry you are, how much you want to eat and how much you weigh.

"Discoveries of complex and interwoven hormone pathways regulating appetite, metabolism, fat production and fat breakdown also suggest a more biological basis for the setpoint," wrote Brian Rowley, MS, in an article on the subject for *Muscle & Fitness Hers* magazine.[4] Respiratory quotient, a measure of how much energy a body burns in a day from carbohydrates versus fats, may also be a factor in setpoints. "People with high respiratory quotients burn proportionately more carbs and conserve fats, while those with low respiratory quotients burn more fats and fewer carbs," writes Rowley. It is those people with the higher quotients that are two-and-a-half times more likely to gain 11 or more pounds in two to four years.

To determine where your weight falls in

relation to your setpoint, ask yourself the following questions:

● At what weight does my body seem most "comfortable?" This isn't necessarily your ideal weight.

● Is there a particular weight my body tends to climb back to after weight loss? If so, what is it?

● What is the most I have ever weighed?

The answers to these questions should give you a good indication of what your setpoint is. While the natural tendency is for people to lose weight and gain it back, there are ways to lower your setpoint. The secret is to weight cycle down to your desired weight when you want to.

How To Lower Your Setpoint

There are two ways of lowering your setpoint to lose weight. You can go on a special ketogenic diet and/or you can exercise. I recommend both.

Step 1: Diet

My premium crash diets, The 10-Days-10-Pounds-Off Program and Dr. Nagler's 500 Diet are ketogenic, low-carbohydrate diets that lower your insulin level and lower your setpoint. You eat less and experience less hunger and, as a result of lowering your setpoint, decrease the percentage of fat that your body is carrying.

An important element of my diet is drinking water. Drinking water is essential. You need to drink enough water to allow your kidneys to dispose of waste products through your urine. If you have an aversion to water, choose no-calorie alternatives like diet soda, coffee or tea.

The reason my crash diets work is that you lose weight fast, which keeps you motivated, so you stay on your diet until you reach your goal. You see results right away and are less likely to lose interest and cheat. On average, you can lose five to 10 pounds your first week and 10-20 pounds every month.

Step 2: Exercise

The more you exercise, the more calories you burn. The more calories you burn, the faster you lose weight. In terms of resetting your setpoint, exercise is essential. Weight training helps change your body composition by building lean muscle tissue and cardiovascular training helps teach your body to use oxygen more efficiently. After about six weeks of regular exercise, your metabolic rate speeds up, so you burn more calories throughout the day. In other words, regular exercise lowers your setpoint. If you cut down on your food intake and exercise, fat-burning increases even more and you lose weight even faster.

If you continue to exercise after you have reached your goal, you can eat more than you used to without gaining weight. Exercise changes your setpoint. In the maintenance portion of this book, I have outlined a weight-training and cardiovascular program that can help you reset your metabolic setpoint and keep your weight off, if you want to.

The problem is that many people don't like physical activity. I recommend that you start exercising slowly, so you get into the habit of moving everyday. For every mile you walk, you burn about 100 calories. Remember, it doesn't matter how quickly you cover the mile in terms of establishing a habit. The distance covered is the key.

Exercise makes you burn more calories and lose weight faster. Get your personal physician's approval first, of course, especially if you are morbidly obese or have heart problems. The more you exercise, the better you will feel. And you'll probably live longer, too. Below you will find my simple exercise program that can help you get into the habit of doing weight training and cardiovascular exercise. It has been designed to be easy to do and not take up a lot of time. Try and complete this workout three times a week. If you want to do more, add time to the cardiovascular portion first, then add another set of exercise repetitions (reps).

The Habit-Forming Workout

Resistance Training:

Exercise	Sets	Reps
Squat	1-3	12-15
Lunge	1-3	12-15
Push-Up	1-3	12-15
Crunch	1-3	12-15

Cardiovascular Training:

Walk 1 mile three times a week. Time yourself. Once you can walk a mile in 15 minutes, increase your distance by 10 percent each week.

Exercise Descriptions

Squat

Stand erect with your knees slightly bent and your feet about hip width apart. Push your hips back as if you were sitting in a chair and bend your knees, bringing your thighs parallel to the ground. (Make sure your knees don't go past your toes). Squeeze your butt as you press back up.

Lunge

With your arms extended by your sides, take a large step forward with your right foot. Keep your head up and back straight. This is your start position. Drop your left leg toward the floor by bending both knees. Make sure your right knee doesn't pass over the plane of your toes. Stop just short of your rear knee touching the ground as your front thigh comes parallel to the floor. Press back up, forcing your body weight through the heel of your forward foot. Complete reps on the right side and then switch to work the left side. As this exercise gets easier, try holding a dumbbell in each hand.

Push-Ups

Start this exercise either on your knees or on your toes. Place your hands just outside your shoulders on the floor with elbows bent at 90 degrees and your upper arms parallel to the floor. Keep your midsection tight and tucked in. Slowly lower your torso while keeping your elbows pointing toward the ceiling. As your face approaches the floor, keep your neck and head in alignment with your body. Extend your arms to push yourself back up.

Crunch

Lie on the floor with your knees bent and hands behind your head. Curl up, bringing you torso toward your knees. Concentrate on crunching your abdominal muscles as you come up. Try to get your shoulder blades off the floor. Don't pull on your head or press your chin into your chest.

How To Stay On A Diet

After a few days on either my 10-Days-10-Pounds-Off Program or Dr. Nagler's 500 Diet, you may need some help to stay motivated. You're allowed to be human. Half of losing weight is making a decision to stay on your diet. It's easy to fall off the wagon. Sara Lee and McDonald's aren't planning to go out of business. Temptation is always going to be there for you. It's hard to impossible to lose weight if you're constantly cheating.

Why is losing weight such a chore? Why is it so hard for most people to stay on a diet long enough and consistently enough to lose weight and keep it off for any significant period of time? The problem is that knowing what you need to do to lose weight isn't enough. Knowing what you need to do to lose weight is not the same thing as doing it.

The Myth Of Low Self-Esteem

It's certainly not self-image that keeps people fat. That's for sure. Studies show that there are just as many skinny people who hate themselves as there are fat people who hate themselves. You could spend the next 12 years on a psychiatrist's couch learning to fall madly in love with yourself and still be overweight. And it's not a matter of motivation or how much you want to lose weight. I don't know anybody on the face of the earth more motivated to lose weight than fat people.

And don't let anyone give you a hard time about willpower. It's not a matter of willpower, it's a matter of insulin level. Overweight people have high insulin levels, which makes it hard to control appetite. When your insulin level is high, you overeat. The more you overeat, the higher your insulin level goes. And over time, rising insulin levels can effect body chemistry to such a degree that it can become extremely difficult to lose weight.

The secret to losing weight is to eat less food than your body needs. You have to find a way to effectively starve yourself. Most people find this extremely difficult. However, some people are brilliant at it. Take thin people, for example. Most thin adults watch their weight. They don't eat everything they want. They hold back. And when they do indulge, they don't get carried away and gain a ton of weight. Thin people watch their intake and take the extra few pounds off — before things get out of hand. Thin people can teach you a lot about weight loss.

The Thin Attitude

Eighteen years ago, I began my first weight-loss study by examining the habits of naturally thin people. I interviewed more than 100 naturally thin people. I wanted to find out how they stayed thin. I wanted to find out how they were different. I had many questions. What was it about thin people's lives, lifestyles, food choices, preferences, hair color or whatever that allowed them to remain thin and in control when it came to food? I wanted to find out how thin people stayed thin, without a struggle. So I asked them.

Me: "Do you ever gain weight?"
Thin Person: "Yes."
Me: "When do you gain weight?"
Thin Person: "After Christmas, New Years, Thanksgiving, vacations, that sort of thing. I put on a few pounds any time I eat too much. If I eat too much popcorn at the movies, or eat too many sweets or go to a party and have too many drinks, I put on a little weight."
Me: "So, what do you do when you want to lose weight?"

Thin Person: "Well, I just stop eating so much."

Me: "OK, but when you want to lose weight, what do you eat?"

Thin Person: "Nothing."

Me: "But specifically, when you want to lose weight, what exactly do you eat?"

Thin Person: "Nothing."

Me: "You don't eat anything when you want to lose weight?"

Thin Person: "Nothing in particular."

Me: "You mean you don't go on a diet to lose weight?"

Thin Person: "No, of course not. I just cut down. I stop eating so much. I don't do anything special."

Me: "But aren't you hungry?"

Thin Person: "Of course, but how else can you lose weight?"

So there it was, staring me in the face. The difference between thin people and fat people was so simple, so obvious, so self-evident and elementary that I had missed it completely. Thin people knew that they have to be hungry in order to lose weight.

They were not looking for the magic "no

hunger" diet. The naturally thin people in my study were realistic. They knew that they had to be hungry to lose weight. So I decided to conduct another study to find out if "being hungry" was the secret to losing weight.

My Study On "Being Hungry"

In my second study, I gathered together 40 overweight people at the University of Michigan League in the spring of 1983. I told my volunteers that I was going to try to help them lose weight with a radical new approach. My volunteers were to work on being hungry. I told them that it was OK not to eat. They were given one single instruction. They were to go without eating whenever they could, for as long as they could. That was it. I would see everyone again in two months.

The results were surprising. When we met again two months later, nobody had lost an ounce. But the shocker was that 20 percent of my volunteers had quit smoking. I suspected I was on to something, but I didn't know what. There's an old saying in psychiatry: "Control in any direction is control." Apparently my instruction to "be hungry" had somehow allowed my smokers to gain enough control over themselves to kick the habit, but not enough control over their appetites to lose any weight.

After thinking about it for a while, it occurred to me that smoking is an easier habit to break than overeating. Smoking is something you don't have to go back to. You can give it up forever. Overeating, on the other hand, is more complicated. It is a matter of degree. You can't give up food entirely. You need food to survive.

So what was it about my study that made it easier for some of my volunteers to quit smoking? All they were told to do was to try to be hungry. The message was loud and clear: It was OK to want food and not eat. Then it occurred to me: Twenty percent of my volunteers made a very powerful generalization. They discovered that it was OK to desire something and not satisfy that desire. In other words, 20 percent learned that it was OK to want a cigarette and not smoke. It sort of made sense.

But, how was this going to help me help people to lose weight? I asked myself what was it about being hungry that was so threatening to an overweight person? What was the big deal about not eating so much? What was the problem? Anxiety, perhaps? I started thinking about flooding, a psychological technique that was used in the 1920s to treat anxiety.

Taking The Anxiety Out Of Weight Loss

The early studies on flooding started with a group of researchers who were experimenting with reptile phobias. The researchers were looking for a way to cure people of a fear of snakes. They had come up with an incredible technique that yielded an astonishing result: total cure in every case. It had never been done before.

The researchers would take an individual who was afraid of snakes. They would do a brief cardiac examination to make sure that the subject had no serious heart or blood pressure problems. Then the researchers would tie the subject down to a secure chair, which was also bolted to the floor. You can guess what happened next. Exactly. The researchers dropped a very large, very slippery, very frightening snake, right in the subject's lap. The screaming would go on anywhere from five minutes to half an hour. The subjects would sweat bullets and plead for mercy. But the torture would not let up. And then suddenly the screaming, sweating and pleading would stop.

It wasn't that each and every subject had died of fright. But rather, the brutal experiment had actually worked. After 30 minutes of torture, each and every subject's fear of snakes completely disappeared. It was fascinating. Most of the subjects began to laugh. They lost their fear completely and the result seemed to be permanent. On a followup study more than a year later, all subjects remained unafraid of snakes. The desensitization process, or flooding as it came to be called, never went away. All subjects tested lost their fear of snakes forever, in just one treatment.

Researchers continued their work on other problems. Total cures were reported again and again. They tried the technique on people who were afraid of heights, dangling subjects by ropes attached to the tops of tall buildings. The same results were reported every time. When the screaming stopped, the volunteers were no longer afraid of heights. They took subjects who were afraid of spiders, strapped them down and dropped large defanged tarantulas on them. When the shouting stopped, the subjects were cured.

Flooding swept through the psychiatric community in the late 1920s and quickly established itself as the treatment of choice to help people overcome specific fears and anxiety. But just as quickly, with the birth of anti-anxiety drugs in the early 1930s, the flooding technique was forgotten.

Thirty years later, science had another breakthrough that stimulated the minds of flooding technique researchers. The invention of EMG or Electromyogram unlocked scientists' ability to measure the electrical activity of muscles. Numerous studies have been performed using EMG to determine muscle stimulation. When researchers hooked up an EMG to a subject's arm and had that person swing a tennis racket or lift a heavy object, they recorded the firing of certain muscles. The researchers then had the same person just think of swinging a tennis racket or lifting a heavy object, without moving. What the EMG studies found was that the very same activity occurred in the very same muscles. Even though the subjects did not move, the muscles fired. These results led to all sorts of interesting hypotheses. Advocates of flooding suggested that perhaps thinking or imagining alone could help people to get rid of their phobias.

The flooding experts wondered what would happen if they didn't use real snakes in flooding therapy. What would happen if they asked their subjects to imagine the snakes instead? What would happen if those who were afraid of heights were asked to just imagine themselves dangling from the top of a tall building? What would happen to arachniphobics if they were asked to imagine spiders crawling up and down their arms? Would just thinking about a phobic object allow subjects to lose their fear of the real thing? The researchers did a number of experiments and the answer came back a resounding "Yes!"

In experiment after experiment, the researchers demonstrated lasting phobia cures without using snakes or tall buildings. Snake phobic subjects imagined a snake in their lap, until they felt like screaming, and the fear of snakes went away. Subjects who were afraid of heights imagined they were dangling from the top of a tall building until they experienced anxiety and their fear of heights went away. The researchers demonstrated the same 100 percent cure rate, using imaginary objects instead of the real thing. The new era in cognitive psychiatry was born and the technique was called implosion therapy.

Implosion Therapy For Weight Loss

I wondered if my volunteers were having difficulty losing weight because they were afraid of being hungry. I decided to test my hypothesis and see if implosion therapy could help decondition their fear of being hungry. I reunited my group of subjects from the University of Michigan and tried implosion to ease anxiety associated with being hungry. I wanted to see if implosion would make it easier for people not to eat.

This time it worked. Seventy-three percent of my subjects lost an average of more than 20 pounds and kept it off for more than a year. Those who lost weight attributed their weight loss to eating less food and being able to experience hunger more easily. Of the treated subjects who didn't lose weight, they stated that they didn't want to be hungry to lose weight. Implosion therapy for weight loss was born. [5]

Implosion therapy works for weight loss because most heavy people experience anxiety when they try not to eat. Fat people don't have an eating disorder. They have a "not eating" disorder. Fat people have no problem eating. They are overly good at it. It's why they are fat.

I've found three different types of implosion therapy to help people lose weight: Positive, Negative and Motivating.

1. Positive Implosion Therapy extinguishes "not eating" anxiety with relaxing, feel-good, eating imagery. It allows you to fantasize about eating all your favorite foods. The idea is that you're less tempted to cheat on your diet, because you've already satisfied your desires.

2. Negative Implosion Therapy is quite different, but very powerful. It extinguishes "not eating" anxiety by using negative imagery to get you off, and keep you off, your problem foods. The technique makes foods you normally find appealing to be disgusting. Negative Implosion Therapy eliminates from your diet the foods you have no business eating in the first place. If you can't stop eating chocolate sundaes, carrot cake, Hershey bars or whatever — Negative Implosion can help you.

3. Motivating Implosion Therapy helps you to stay on your diet. It acts like a cheerleader. It keeps you focused, dieting and feeling good about yourself as you lose weight. Motivating Implosion takes the struggle out of dieting so you aren't tempted to deviate from your weight-loss program.

From my research, some people respond better to Positive Implosion, while others do better with Negative Implosion. I've found what works best for most people is to start with both the Positive and Negative Implosion imagery. Over the course of a week, you'll find yourself gravitating more toward one technique or the other. Go with the one that works best for you.

The Positive and Negative Implosion techniques used for dieting are divided into two sections: sweets and starches. Sweets and starches are the typical foods that cause problems for people when they go on a diet. Let's say you tend to get in trouble with sweet foods like ice cream. Every time you try to lose weight, after a few days of successful dieting, you find yourself hitting your local ice cream store. Or maybe it's not ice cream that's the trouble. Perhaps it's chocolate chip cookies or candy. For others, starches cause the most grief. Trying to go without bagels or pizza is too much to bear. Or saying no to potato chips is virtually impossible.

Making Implosion Therapy Work For You

Implosion Therapy can help you get rid of your cravings for sweets and starches. You'll need a friend to read the implosion imagery to you or a tape recorder to record the imagery yourself. (You can also order the tapes I use from www.dietresults.com or by calling 1-800-511-9769. The tapes are produced in recorded loops so you only have to rewind once a week.)

From my experience, half a dozen foods cause trouble for most dieters. Make a list of your problem foods. Pick one to start with. Once this problem food is under control, which takes about a week for most people, move on to the next troublemaker on your list. And so on.

Appendix 2 contains my scripts for Positive, Negative and Motivating Implosion. There are Positive and Negative Implosions for the most common problem foods. Your problem food should be covered. If it's not, make the appropriate substitutions in the script. Record both the Positive and Negative Implosions for your problem foods. Record the Motivating

Implosion. Speak slowly and succinctly. Your implosion tape should run about two to three minutes.

To keep you dieting, do one session of Positive or Negative Implosion once a day, followed by Motivating Implosion. Listen to your tapes whenever you have the time. It will take you less than five minutes. Five minutes a day isn't much to ask to keep you on track.

It doesn't matter when you do the implosion. You can listen to the tapes first thing in the morning, late at night, during your lunch break or whenever. Take a five-minute break when you are someplace where you can close your eyes. Follow the instructions and run through the imagery in your mind. Don't listen to the tape while you are driving. You need to be able to give 100 percent of your attention to the implosion to have it work for you. Besides, I don't want you driving and imploding with your eyes closed at the same time.

Within a few days, you'll get a sense of whether you respond better to Positive or Negative Implosion. Stick to the one that works best for you. After about a week, when your problem food is under control, pick another food on your list. Try both the Positive and Negative Implosion imagery for the second food item. You may find that a different implosion technique works better this time. Cravings for some foods will extinguish better with Positive Implosion. Other foods do better with the Negative technique. In either case, it usually takes about a week to get most foods under control. After you have completed Positive or Negative Implosion on your half-dozen problem foods, just do a Motivating Implosion session once a day to keep you focused and crash dieting.

Section 2:

Dr. Nagler's Crash Diets

Crash Diet Instructions

Follow these rules exactly. You can lose five to 10 pounds your first week and four to five pounds every week thereafter. You CANNOT cheat or deviate from these guidelines. Follow my instructions carefully and you will feel at your best on my crash diets.

1) If You're Not Hungry, Don't Eat

If you want to lose weight as rapidly as possible on the 10-Days-10-Pounds-Off Program or my 500 Diet, the most important thing to remember is this: *If you're not hungry, don't eat.* I'll say it again. I can't emphasize it enough: *If you're not hungry, don't eat.*

Don't have breakfast or anything at all if you're not hungry. The less you eat, the faster you will lose weight.

It's as simple as that. If you're not hungry, don't eat. There's no magic. The less you eat, the faster you will lose weight. After two to three days you'll be in the fat-burning state of ketosis (See Section 1) on either diet, so you will not be particularly hungry. Not eating will be a lot easier than it sounds.

2) Drink Water

You have to drink water. You have to drink at least 128 ounces of water every day. This means you must drink about 12 10-ounce glasses of water (or other non-caloric fluid) every day. Drinking 150-200 ounces a day is even better. You need this much fluid to flush out the fat you are burning and keep your kidneys healthy.

Water is the healthiest thing to drink, but coffee, tea, Diet Coke and diet sodas are fine. You don't have to drink water at all if you hate it. Most people find that once they get into the habit of drinking water, they love it. Remember, you must drink at least 128 ounces of non-caloric fluid a day to lose weight and feel at your best on my crash diets.

You will be in ketosis, so you really need to push fluids to flush out the fat you are burning. On ketogenic diets (See Section 1) like my 10-Days-10-Pounds-Off Program and my 500 Diet, you are expelling fat through your urine. Drinking water is absolutely imperative. You do not want to get dehydrated or stress your kidneys. Once you are in ketosis, you can drink Diet

Snapple or Crystal Lite, but only if you check your urine with Ketostix every time you urinate. If you can remain in ketosis drinking Diet Snapple and Crystal Lite, drink them. If not, throw them away. Absolutely NO regular soda or sugared drinks are allowed!

It's almost impossible to drink too much water or fluid on my program. The more you drink the better you will do and the better you will feel. Try to drink your weight in ounces of water. For example, if you weigh 150 pounds, try to drink at least 150 ounces of water every day. If you weigh 250 pounds, try to drink at least 250 ounces of water a day. Check with your doctor who is supervising you to determine how much water is good for you. It is possible to dilute the amount of sodium and potassium in your blood by over-hydrating, but this is very rare.

3) Get Into Ketosis

When you are in ketosis, you are burning fat at a very high rate. The best way to get your body into ketosis quickly and speed up weight loss on any of my programs is to eat only the protein list for two to three days. If you are very hungry, you may have a third serving of protein while you are getting into ketosis. Do not have anything else. NO fruit, vegetables or salads — nothing else until you are in ketosis. Then follow the crash diets exactly as written. This applies to all my crash diets except for the 10-Days-10-Pounds-Off Program, which requires that you eat a 1/2 grapefruit before every meal.

To check if you are in ketosis, use Ketostix, which can be purchased at any drugstore or from www.dietresults.com. Dip the colored end of a Ketostix strip in a fresh urine specimen or pass it through a stream of urine. After 15 seconds, compare the color of the end of the Ketostix with the color chart on the side of the Ketostix bottle. If your strip is medium pink, you are in small or moderate ketosis, which is where you want to be. If the strip shows pale pink or beige, you are not in ketosis. If you are not in ketosis, eliminate all carbohydrates from your diet. If the strip shows medium or dark purple, you are dehydrated. Drink more water immediately. Check your urine with Ketostix every time you urinate.

4) Use Equal and Sweet 'N Low Tablets Only (No Packets), No Flavored Coffee, No Creamer

You may add Equal or Sweet 'N Low tablets to your coffee or tea if you need a sweetener. But NO Equal or Sweet 'N Low packets. The packets contain more carbohydrates than the tablets and can knock you out of ketosis and trigger feelings of hunger. To get into the quick fat-burning state of ketosis, you will be drastically limiting your carbohydrate intake. Absolutely no flavored coffees, coffee creamers, coffee whitener or cappuccino. Their carbohydrate content is way too high for my crash diets. Even a little extra carbohydrate can quickly knock you out of ketosis and stop you from losing weight.

You may have only diet drinks that are zero calorie AND zero carbohydrate. That means you can drink all the canned or bottled diet soda (Diet Coke, Diet 7-Up, Diet Dr Pepper, etc.) you can down. No other diet drinks are allowed on my 10-Days-10-Pounds-Off Program or Dr. Nagler's 500 Diet. Any sweetener or drink with more than a zero calorie and zero carbohydrate count is off limits. Given that I am asking you to drink a lot of fluids, minute amounts of carbohydrates can really add up in drinks with 1 gram of carbohydrate. Stay away from powdered sweeteners and powdered diet drinks. Your carbohydrate intake can rapidly get out of control.

5) No Breath Mints Or Gum Allowed Until You Are In Ketosis

Once you are in ketosis, you can chew sugarless gum and use sugarless breath mints, but only if you check your urine with Ketostix and can remain in ketosis after using them. For bad breath it's best to take three Breath Asure capsules every two to three hours. Breath Asure can be purchased by calling 800-511-9769 and from www.dietresults.com.

6) Constipation And The Apple Diet

You can rarely experience mild constipation on either of my crash diets. Little is going in, so very little may come out. If you are constipated, take a day off and with your doctor's permission go on my Apple Diet. On the Apple Diet you eat six apples a day

— and that's it. You can't have anything else other than your 128 ounces of water. Make sure that you are drinking your water to help this extra fiber push through your system. Otherwise, you can feel bloated and cramped. If constipation persists throughout the course of this program, consult your doctor.

7) **Finally, unless your doctor says otherwise, don't stay on my 10-Days-10-Pounds-Off Program or Dr. Nagler's 500 Diet for more than 2 months.** Remember, please don't go on any of my programs without medical supervision.

Helpful Hints To Guarantee Success

Follow your diet. Eat the foods from your food list only. Follow all of my instructions exactly. If at any time you are not hungry, don't eat. The less you eat, the faster you will lose weight. You do not have to finish everything on your plate or eat three meals a day. If a food is not mentioned, you can't have it.

Drink water. Drink at least 128 ounces of water a day. In addition, you may have as much coffee, tea, sparkling water and diet soda as you want. If you get hungry, drink a glass of non-caloric liquid before you eat anything. You may find that your hunger fades.

Avoid fat and sugar. Try to completely eliminate all butter, margarine, fat and oil from your diet. Avoid sugar and honey like the plague. Read labels carefully when you go shopping to avoid unwanted sugar (carbohydrate) and fat.

Move. Exercise is always recommended

for weight loss. Try to get in the habit of walking for 20 minutes, four to five times a week. This can provide a habit that you can carry into your maintenance plan. Exercise can help keep your weight off for a longer period of time.

Master the art of ordering. Almost a third of all meals are eaten away from home. You need to know how to eat in restaurants while on a diet without feeling deprived. You shouldn't feel like you are being tortured just because you are dining out. You are paying good money for a good time.

Ask for what you want. Ask for your food to be prepared dry, without butter, margarine or oil. Ask for your food to be broiled, baked, steamed or poached. Ask for all sauces and dressings on the side. Ask for low-fat and low-carbohydrate sauces and dressings. Ask for mustard, lemon juice, horseradish and hot sauce to add flavor.

Restaurants provide a service — cooking. You're paying quite a bit for this service. Have it your way. Be polite. Wait and kitchen staff are more apt to fulfill special requests nowadays and they are even happier when the person asking is respectful and courteous. This way you are more likely to get exactly what you want.

What can you order when you are dining out? Anything that used to walk, swim, fly, run or crawl — cooked without butter, margarine or oil. Order fish dry and put lemon on it. Have two or three shrimp cocktails. Order an omelet made with EggBeaters or with four egg whites and one yolk. Have a steamed or broiled lobster. Have a hamburger without the bun. Have a scoop of tuna made with no-fat mayonnaise.

If you're out for lunch or dinner, and you have to eat something, eating the foods on this list, will keep you in ketosis. You're better off staying exactly on my 10-Days-10-Pounds-Off or my 500 Diet, but this list is your fallback.

Desperation Dining-Out Choices

Quiche or pizza — no crust

Fajita — no tortilla, no guacamole, no sour cream

Roll-up sandwich — made with lettuce, not bread

Kabob — beef or chicken, no rice

Egg white or EggBeaters omelet

Salad — Cobb, Greek, Chef, Grilled Chicken; use low-fat or fat-free dressing

Shrimp cocktail

Fish — poached, steamed, broiled, grilled; cooked with no fat

Shellfish — poached, steamed, broiled, grilled; cooked with no fat

String cheese — low-fat or fat-free

Beef jerky — no brown sugar

Hot dog or Vienna sausage — no bun

Tuna — made with lemon juice or fat-free mayonnaise

Arby's roast beef — no bun

Burger King — hamburger/broiled chicken, no bun, salad with low-fat dressing

Wendy's — hamburger/broiled chicken, no bun, salad with low-fat dressing

Boston Market — chicken no skin

McDonald's — hamburger/broiled chicken, no bun, salad with low-fat dressing

There Are No Calories In Christmas, Easter or Thanksgiving. There are no calories in your birthday, anniversary or graduation, either. Why do people put on weight during the holidays and special occasions? The reason is simple. You increase your intake of fat. You eat too much cake or too many chips. You constantly have your hands in the candy bowl. You pile on the gravy and have to have a second helping of Grandma's potatoes. You go to parties and eat when you aren't hungry.

Avoid putting on holiday pounds by watching your intake of fat. Keep your portions small. You can still enjoy holiday goodies with your friends and family. Just make the right choices. Choose one dessert instead of two or three, and don't eat the whole thing. Just take a bite or two. There's no rule that says that you have to lick your plate clean. There is no need to try everything. You know what most of it tastes like anyway.

The other high-caloric trap of the holidays is alcohol. Alcohol is the Great Enabler as far as dieting is concerned. Alcohol stimulates the appetite and is also high in calories. During the holidays, it can be hard to abstain. You may have one drink or one dessert, not both. Have whichever you want. Have exactly what you want. For example, if you want white wine, don't settle for red. If you want chocolate ice cream, don't settle for vanilla. This way you'll be more satisfied with less of what you chose. As the saying goes: "You can never get enough of what you really don't want."

Frequently Asked Questions

Don't I need to eat something to keep my metabolism burning?

Absolutely not. Your body metabolism is always burning whether you eat or not. Your metabolism does not significantly slow down or speed up throughout the day unless you are exercising, which gives your metabolism a bit of a push.

I'm craving sweets. What should I do?

If you have sweet cravings, stop all chicken, turkey, eggs, EggBeaters and cottage cheese for two or three days. Your sweet cravings should go away. Poultry and dairy products are loaded with hormones that can make you crave sweets.

What can I do about my dry mouth?

Drink more water! If you are drinking your 128 ounces of water a day, dry mouth should not be a problem. If you are drinking at least a gallon of water a day and your mouth is still dry, try 500mg-1500mg Evening Primrose capsules, one to three times a day.

What can I do about my bad breath?

Try Breath Asure, three capsules every three or four hours. Drink eight to 12 ounces of water each time you take the capsules and your breath will be fine. Remember to stay away from sugarless gum and breath mints, which kick you out of ketosis and can stop you from losing weight.

Why do I have to drink so much water?

You need to drink at least 128 ounces of water a day (in addition to all the coffee, tea and diet soda you want) to flush out all the fat you are burning and to avoid damage to your kidneys.

Can I drink diet soda instead of water?

Yes, if you can't stand water. But remember you must always drink at least 128 ounces of non-caloric fluid a day.

What can I eat for breakfast?

Before you even think about eating, drink at least a quart of non-caloric fluid, preferably water. If you are still hungry, then eat from your food list. Eat only from your food list, and eat as little as possible. You want to save the bulk of your daily calories for later in the day when real hunger usually sets in.

What can I do to lose weight faster?

If you're not hungry, don't eat! Pay attention to whether you are hungry or not. Avoid recreational eating or grazing. Unless you are truly hungry, don't eat. Keep drinking your water.

I'm not in ketosis. What's wrong?

You're probably eating too many carbohydrates. Eat only from your meat list. Stop all fruits and vegetables. Make sure you are drinking your water. You should be in ketosis in one or two days.

I can't sleep. Is something wrong?

Stop all caffeine (Diet Coke, coffee and tea). Make sure that you are drinking at least 128 ounces of water a day.

Will eating so much protein raise my cholesterol?

Serum cholesterol is determined more by the fat stored in your body than by the fat in your diet. When you lose weight, you

lose stored fat, which helps lower your cholesterol. When you first start a high protein
diet, your cholesterol will rise a bit. But as
you begin to lose weight, your cholesterol
will fall.

Dr. Nagler's 10-Days-10-Pounds-Off Program

This is the most popular diet in my office and the one you should go on with your doctor's permission, especially if you like grapefruit. Read through the menu below and follow my instructions exactly. Always remember: If you're not hungry, don't eat.

BREAKFAST
1/2 Grapefruit
Coffee or Tea

If you're hungry, start your day with a 1/2 grapefruit, and as much black coffee or plain tea as you like and can get down. However, for the umpteenth time, if you're not hungry, don't eat.

Coffee and Tea

There's magic in the caffeine in coffee, tea and Diet Coke. Caffeinated beverages can help you feel better, give you a caffeine-induced energy high and help burn fat faster. Caffeine can increase levels of cyclic adenosine monophosphate (cAMP), which can result in the liberation of free fatty acids from fat cells.[6] This can make you feel like you have more energy. If you're caffeine-sensitive or caffeine doesn't make you feel good, don't have any. If caffeine keeps you up at night, switch to decaffeinated beverages after noon or whatever your personal cut-off time is.

You may not have creamer or whitener or skim milk or anything in your coffee or tea. If you must drink your coffee white, add my vanilla formula, available by calling 800-511-9769 and www.dietresults.com. Use Equal or Sweet 'N Low tablets only, not the powdered packets. The packets contain too much hidden carbohydrate and can throw you out of ketosis and slow your weight loss.

You also don't have to drink Diet Coke. My brother prefers Diet Pepsi. I don't care what you drink, as long as it's non-caloric and preferably caffeinated. Incidentally, Diet Mountain Dew has about the highest caffeine content of any of the diet sodas.

Grapefruit

You must eat a 1/2 grapefruit before any meal. You don't have to eat all of the food or meals on the list, but you must have the 1/2 grapefruit before eating anything else. If you are hungry in between meals, you may also have a 1/2 grapefruit as a snack. Eat no more than three whole grapefruit a day. If you want your grapefruit sweeter, add one Equal or Sweet 'N Low packet to your grapefruit. If you're eating out and grapefruit isn't on the menu, you're out of luck. Carry a grapefruit with you and pay the restaurant a plating fee to serve you half. Ask them to wrap up the other half so you can take it home with you. Grapefruit juice is not allowed.

Grapefruit provides bulk and fiber, satisfies your sweet cravings and makes you feel full. There's no metabolic magic or fat-burning secret to eating grapefruit before each meal, despite the selection of grapefruit "fat-burning" tablets you can buy at most health-food stores. However, recent research released out of the Scripps Clinic at the University of San Diego on Jan. 26, 2004, showed that grapefruit can influence fat loss.

Scientists studied 100 men and women who were divided into three groups. One ate 1/2 a grapefruit with each meal, a second drank eight ounces of grapefruit juice three times a day and a third acted as a control group. All groups maintained their regular eating habits during the course of the study. Despite the fact that none of the subjects actually dieted during a 12-week period, the average weight loss in both the grapefruit and grapefruit juice groups was about four pounds. Several subjects reported losing 10 or more pounds[7].

Despite this finding, drinking juice of any kind — grapefruit, orange, tomato, carrot, etc. — is completely off limits. Drinking juice is one of the best ways I know to gain a whole bunch of weight in a hurry. Take grapefruit juice for example. A big glass of sweetened grapefruit juice usually contains well in excess of 200 calories, and probably takes less than a minute to drink. On the other hand, one half of a very large grapefruit usually contains less than 50 calories, and takes most people three to five minutes to eat. Think about it. If you ate as many grapefruit halves to equal the calories in a single glass of grapefruit juice (I'm talking about two whole grapefruit here), it would take you close to 20 minutes, and you'd probably be sick to your stomach to boot.

LUNCH
1/2 Grapefruit
Salad (up to 2 cups)
Omelet made with EggBeaters OR 4 Egg
Whites, 1 Egg Yolk and Bacos
Coffee or Tea

If you are not hungry for lunch, for goodness sake don't eat. If you are hungry, start lunch the same way you start every other meal you eat on this program — with a 1/2 grapefruit. After your grapefruit, if you are satisfied and no longer hungry, stop eating.

If you are still hungry after your 1/2 grapefruit, you can go on to the rest of the meal. Once again, if your hunger is satisfied after you have your 1/2 grapefruit, stop eating. You don't have to eat the salad or the omelet. If you are hungry, go ahead and eat!

Salad
While on this diet it is important that you do not shy away from the vegetables. Not only do vegetables provide you with a host of vitamins and minerals that keep you healthy, vegetables provide fiber that keeps

you feeling full and that keeps you regular. You can eat two salads a day, one at lunch and another at dinner.

Both lunch and dinner salads have a maximum total volume of 2 cups each. Salad consists only of the following vegetables in any combination:

● Lettuce (Darker greens like romaine and mesclun have more nutrients and fiber.)
● Cucumbers
● Mushrooms
● Onions
● Radishes
● Sprouts

NO carrots, tomatoes, or any other vegetables. NO cheese or croutons. You may use up to 2 tablespoons of a low-fat, low-carbohydrate dressing on your salad. Look for a dressing that has no more than 3 grams of fat and no more than 3 grams of carbohydrate per single serving.

Omelet Made With EggBeaters OR 4 Egg Whites, 1 Egg Yolk And Bacos

Lunch consists of a small container of EggBeaters (one 4-ounce carton) or one whole egg and three egg whites, lightly scrambled or served as an omelet. Cook in a nonstick pan with butter-flavored PAM, Butterbuds or your favorite fat-free butter substitute. Do not use butter, oil or margarine to prepare your eggs or egg substitute. Use all of the herbs and spices you like. If you retain water, are hypertensive or need to watch sodium intake, take it easy on the salt. You may add one heaping tablespoon of Bacos to your scrambled EggBeaters or egg whites, either mixed into the egg mixture before or after cooking.

This is an easy meal to have in a restaurant. Order EggBeaters and one tablespoon of the bacon bits used on salads. Or have them make you an omelet with four egg whites and one egg yolk, along with bacon bits if you want it. Another option is to order four hardboiled eggs, and eat the four whites and just one of the yolks. Of course, you can always leave out the yolk entirely. The yolk is mostly fat and contains 90 percent of the calories of an egg.

DINNER
1/2 Grapefruit
Salad (up to 2 cups)
Vegetable (up to 1 cup)

Meat (up to 8 ounces)
Coffee or Tea

Vegetables

For your vegetables at dinner, you may have up to 1 cup of one of the following vegetables, steamed, roasted or raw, without butter, margarine or oil of any kind:

- Asparagus
- Broccoli
- Brussels sprouts
- Cauliflower
- Mushrooms
- Sauerkraut
- Spinach
- String beans

Enjoy these vegetables without butter or dressing, which adds unwanted calories. Top your vegetable with butter-flavored PAM, Butterbuds or your favorite fat-free butter substitute. Lemon juice is OK, too.

Meat

You may have up to 8 ounces of only one of the following dinner proteins per day:

- Chicken
- Clams
- Crab

- Fish (any type)
- Lobster
- Mussels
- Sardines
- Scallops
- Shrimp
- Turkey
- Veal
- Water-packed tuna

Cooking Directions: Broil, bake, roast, steam or pan fry your protein in a nonstick pan, without butter, margarine or oil. Season with salt, pepper, soy sauce, ketchup, lemon juice, mustard or cocktail sauce. Use no oil, no butter, no margarine, no breading on anything. Lemon juice, mustard and vinegar are OK.

Dessert

If you're absolutely going out of your mind for something sweet, you can have ONE of the following:
- One prepackaged, individual-size serving of sugar-free Jello topped with no more than one tablespoon of fat-free Cool Whip
- One sugar-free Popsicle

- One sugar-free Fudgesicle
- One sugar-free Creamsicle

You can have only one, not one of each. I am not recommending any of these desserts as a regular occurrence while you are on the program. But if you are feeling desperate, they will not totally kill your progress. Just don't make a habit of them.

MAKING IT EASIER

Most people can lose up to 10 pounds in 10 days on my 10-Days-10-Pounds-Off Program. It is super easy with terrific results. But like anything difficult that you decide to undertake, sometimes it is nice to know how to get through the difficult times. Use these two tips to help you:

(1) **Any time you think you are hungry, drink a 12-ounce glass of water.** Your hunger will likely disappear. Studies show that up to 80 percent of the time people chose to eat, they are thirsty, not hungry.

(2) **Any time you are still hungry after a glass of water, eat another half of a grapefruit.** This means that in addition to

the 1/2 grapefruit you eat before each meal, you can also have up to an additional three halves of grapefruit each day, anytime you are hungry. In other words, you can have up to a total of three whole grapefruit each day if you are hungry. This three grapefruit-a-day total, includes your halves before meals.

Do not postpone your before-meal serving of grapefruit until after a meal. The grapefruit half BEFORE each meal is important because it may satisfy your hunger enough so that you won't want to eat anything else, which is the whole idea in the first place.

Dr. Nagler's 10-Days-10-Pounds-Off Program Summary

BREAKFAST
1/2 Grapefruit
Coffee or Tea

LUNCH
1/2 Grapefruit
Salad (2 cups)
Omelet made with EggBeaters OR 4 Egg
Whites, 1 Egg Yolk and Bacos
Coffee or Tea

DINNER
1/2 Grapefruit
Salad (2 cups)
Vegetable (1 cup)
Meat (8 ounces)
Coffee or Tea

Salad with 2 Tbsp. low-fat, low-carbo-hydrate dressing
- Lettuce (Darker greens like romaine and mesclun have more nutrients and fiber.)
- Cucumbers
- Mushrooms

- Onions
- Radishes
- Sprouts

Vegetables
- Asparagus
- Broccoli
- Brussels sprouts
- Cauliflower
- Mushrooms
- Sauerkraut
- Spinach
- String beans

Meat
- Chicken
- Clams
- Crab
- Fish (any type)
- Lobster
- Mussels
- Sardines
- Scallops
- Shrimp
- Turkey
- Veal
- Water-packed tuna

1 — Get your doctor's approval first.

2 — No alcohol or coffee creamer.

3 — Drink 128 ounces of water or non-caloric beverage each day.

4 — No breading, butter, margarine or oil.

5 — Don't eat anything else.

Dr. Nagler's 500 Diet

Dr. Nagler's 500 Diet is my second most popular crash diet. It's ideal for people who eat out a lot and don't want to advertise they are on a diet, and for people who just can't imagine eating all the grapefruit on my 10-Days-10-Pounds-Off Program.

This diet is very low in fat, calories and carbohydrates. It is approximately a 500-calorie diet. The program is designed to make you drop anywhere from one-half pound to a whole pound each day. You will be in ketosis, an accelerated fat-burning state (See page 25), two or three days into the program. This is a very rapid weight-loss program. You will experience accelerated fat burning and an increased level of energy. You really need to push fluid to flush out the fat you are burning and to feel at your best. Keep your water or fluid intake up to at least a gallon (128 ounces) a day. You should feel terrific and lose weight very, very rapidly on this program.

Dr. Nagler's 500 Diet consists of two meals a day, eaten whenever you want. Each meal consists of a meat, a vegetable, a fruit and a drink from the lists. You don't have to eat all of the food, but the meals have been designed to make you feel satisfied. There isn't breakfast or lunch or dinner on this program. You just eat up to two servings of a permitted meat, up to two servings of a permitted fruit and up to two servings of a permitted vegetable every day. For example, if you are hungry when you wake up in morning, you can have an apple and a cup of coffee for breakfast. At lunch, you can have a salad with diet dressing and chicken, and for dinner you can have a piece of fish and some spinach followed by a dessert of six strawberries and coffee. Remember, if you're not hungry, don't eat. You can skip an entire meal, or just eat the meat or fruit or whatever. Just don't have more than two servings of any category. The less you eat, the faster you will lose weight. Whether you eat or not, you must drink at least 128 ounces of non-caloric fluid every day. Drink as much water, coffee, tea and diet soda as you can.

Food can be eaten right out of the can or simply cooked — steamed, boiled, broiled or grilled — without any oil, butter, margarine or fat. Use fat-free mayonnaise or fat-free salad dressing, salt, pepper, relish, garlic, onion salt and any spice (without sugar) you like. Carry a plastic fork and a can opener in your purse or briefcase and you're in business.

Meat

You may have one 4-6 ounce serving of any the following meats up to twice a day. All canned meats must be packed in water, broth, tomato sauce or mustard, NOT oil. Once again, you cannot have canned meat in oil. The easiest and best way to follow the program is to use canned meats because of the built-in portion control.

If you prefer, you can also prepare fresh meats. But if you do, you must weigh your portion before cooking. Better yet, have your butcher or fishmonger divide your meat or fish into individual 4-6 ounce packages. How much you eat is important on this quick weight-loss program.

You can add 1 tablespoon of Miracle Whip Free and 1 teaspoon of pickle relish to each serving of a meat or salad. You may also have unlimited salt, pepper, ketchup, mustard, cocktail sauce and lemon juice. If you are hypertensive, retain water or need to watch your sodium intake, take it easy on the salt. Low-fat or fat-free cheese is not allowed. The reason is that small quantities of fat-free cheeses are not very satisfying, so portion control is difficult. The same is true for lunch meats (beef, pork or poultry). Lunch meats are also way too high in fat and salt. Again, NO low-fat cheese, NO fat-free cheese and NO lunch meats.

Remember, you may have one serving, up to twice a day, of one of the following meats (4-6 ounces per serving unless otherwise indicated):

- Chicken
- Clams
- Cottage cheese (fat-free, 3/4 cup)
- Crab
- EggBeaters (4 ounces)
- Hot dogs (2 fat-free)
- Lobster
- Mussels
- Sardines (packed in water, not oil)
- Shrimp
- Tuna (packed in water, not oil)

- Turkey
- Veal
- Yogurt (1 cup fat-free, 100 calories)

Vegetables

You can have one 8-ounce serving (1 cup) of a vegetable from the following list, up to twice a day. You will do better if you use canned vegetables since the amount you eat on this very rapid weight-loss program is most important. You can get into trouble by exceeding portion size, so be careful when you do your cooking and preparation. A good tip to help keep your portion sizes in check is to leave the grocery store with the vegetables weighed out in 8-ounce portions. This will help you stay in control on the program. I'm sure you want to lose five to 10 pounds your first week and five pounds every week thereafter.

Instead of the 8 ounces of canned or fresh vegetables, you may have 2 cups total volume of a salad instead, consisting of any combination of only the following: lettuce, cucumbers, onions, mushrooms, radishes and sprouts. You may top your salad with one serving (2 tablespoons) of a low-fat, low-carbohydrate dressing containing no more than 3 grams of fat and no more than 3 grams of carbohydrate per serving. NO carrots, tomatoes, potatoes, peas, corn, acorn or any orange-fleshed squash, parsnips or sweet potatoes. These vegetables are way too high in calories and carbohydrates for this very quick weight-loss program.

Remember, you can have one 8-ounce serving (1 cup) of these vegetables, twice a day:

- Asparagus
- Broccoli
- Brussels sprouts
- Cabbage
- Cauliflower
- Celery
- Collard greens
- Cucumbers
- Green beans
- Kale
- Lettuce
- Mushrooms
- Onions
- Peppers (red or green)
- Radishes

- Rutabaga
- Spaghetti squash
- Spinach
- String beans
- Sprouts
- Summer squash
- Swiss chard
- Turnips
- Wax beans
- Zucchini

Use lemon juice, soy sauce, Tabasco sauce, onion powder, garlic, dried spice, salt and pepper to season your vegetables. Be careful with the stronger seasonings that can leave a lingering effect in the mouth. You may be tempted to overeat to get rid of the sensation. Also, if you need to watch your sodium intake, take it easy on the salt.

Fruit
You can have one serving of fruit up to twice a day. The fruit must be fresh, not dried, not canned and not frozen. Do not eat more than two servings of fruit a day. Do not eat fruit that is not on this list. Too

much fruit will stop your weight loss from being as fast as possible.

You may do best on the program if you stick to a 1/2 grapefruit for your fruit. From my clinical experience during the past 20 years with thousands of weight-loss patients, grapefruit seems to work best on the 500 Diet. For many patients, you may be far less hungry if you chose a 1/2 grapefruit for your two fruit servings. If you can't hack grapefruit or it's not available, switch to one of the other fruits on the list. Strawberries are a good second choice. Cantaloupe is a good third.

The reason that I suggest you eat grapefruit while on this diet is that grapefruit provides bulk and fiber, satisfies your sweet cravings and makes you feel full. Drinking juice of any kind — grapefruit, orange, tomato, carrot, etc. — is completely off limits.

You may have 1 fruit, up to twice a day, from the following list:

- 1 apple
- 1/2 cantaloupe
- 1/2 grapefruit

- 12 grapes
- 1 orange
- 6 strawberries

No pears, no cherries, no pineapple, no bananas, no peaches, no figs, no dried and no canned fruit. These fruits are way too high in sugar, calories and carbohydrates for this very quick weight-loss program. Fruits not on the list may stop your weight loss completely.

Please don't eat more than two servings of fruit a day. Don't exceed the recommended portion size and eat only the fruits on my list.

Drink

You have got to push fluid on this diet. Drink at least 128 ounces every day of any of the following:

- Water
- Sugar-free diet soda
- Coffee
- Tea

I have put water first on the list. There's a

good reason for this. I want you to drink as much water as you can first. When you're sick of water, then drink the other recommended beverages. Make sure you drink 128 ounces of non-caloric fluid every day.

Pay attention to the way you feel after drinking coffee, tea and caffeinated beverages (Diet Coke, etc.). Caffeine can trigger hunger and sweet cravings in some people. If caffeine triggers sweet cravings for you, or if you are caffeine sensitive, switch to caffeine-free Diet Coke, decaffeinated coffee, etc.

Remember, no juice, no milk and no regular soda.

Remember:
● Get your personal physician's permission first.
● NO alcoholic beverages or coffee creamer/whitener.
● Use Sweet 'N Low or Equal TABLETS only (NO powdered packets).
● You must drink at least 4 quarts (128 ounces) of water every day.

Dr. Nagler's 500 Diet Summary

Eat one meal twice a day.

Each meal consists of meat, vegetable and fruit.

If you prefer fresh food and want to cook, weigh everything before you eat it.

Canned meats and vegetables are faster and easier.

Meat: One 4-6 ounce serving of:
chicken, clams, crab, lobster, mussels, sardines, shrimp, tuna or turkey.

Vegetable: One 8-ounce water-packed can or 1 cup of:
asparagus, broccoli, brussels sprouts, cauliflower, mushrooms, sauerkraut, spinach or string beans.

Fruit: Fresh only (not canned):
1 apple, 1/2 cantaloupe, 12 grapes, 1/2 grapefruit, 1 orange or 6 strawberries.

1 — Get your doctor's approval first.

2 — No alcohol or creamers.

3 — No lozenges, gum or mints.

4 — Only Breath Asure or Binaca spray.

5 — Sweet 'N Low/Equal tablets only.

6 — Drink four quarts (128 ounces) of water every day.

7 — Don't eat anything else.

Other Crash Diets

If either my 10-Days-10-Pounds-Off Program or Dr. Nagler's 500 Diet is not for you, I have three other crash diets for you to choose from. You will still lose weight quickly.

The key is to pick one diet and stick to it for at least three to four days. Then you can switch to another option, which you also must stick to for three to four days. You should lose 5-10 pounds your first week on all of these programs and about five pounds every week thereafter.

Here are your options:

Dr. Nagler's Very Low-Fat Ketogenic Diet is my easiest program for restaurant eating.

Dr. Nagler's Ketogenic Crash is a super-speedy weight-loss program, if you are good about portion control.

Dr. Nagler's Rotation is designed for those who like a lot of variety and have the discipline to switch diet programs every three to four days.

Option 1: Dr. Nagler's Very Low-Fat Ketogenic Diet

This is my extremely low-fat, semi-free-feeding alternative that's almost as fast as my 10-Days-10-Pounds-Off Program or Dr. Nagler's 500 Diet. It's easy to follow if you eat out a lot. No one will know you are on a diet unless you tell them. You should lose about a pound a day your first week on this program and three to five pounds every week thereafter.

The hardest thing about my Very Low-Fat Ketogenic program is portion control. You may not have more than a normal restaurant-size serving of protein and salad. If you go over normal restaurant-size portions, you won't lose weight anywhere near as fast as you will on the 10-Days-10-Pounds-Off Diet or Dr. Nagler's 500 Diet. Normal restaurant size portions are generally 8 ounces for protein such as meat, fish and poultry, and one to two cups for salad. Do not exceed these portion sizes. You may have up to three servings of meat and up to two servings of salad every day.

For the first two or three days, eat only

lean meat, poultry, fish, seafood and eggs. This will put your body into a ketosis. Check your urine with Ketostix three times a day. Once you are in ketosis, you can add the salad to your diet, but only if you are hungry. This is a very rapid weight-loss program.

PROTEIN
Eat only from the protein list until you are in ketosis. You may have one 4-8 ounce serving of protein up to three times a day.

Lean Meat
Steak, prime rib, hamburgers, pork chops, ribs, lamb chops, veal, hot dogs. Remove all fat before cooking and eating.

Poultry
Chicken, turkey, duck, goose, game hen, ground turkey burgers, turkey hot dogs. No skin.

Fish
Salmon, tuna, swordfish, flounder, grouper, haddock, halibut, cod, scrod, orange roughy, sole, seabass, turbot, monk-

fish. Steamed, boiled, broiled, grilled with no butter, margarine or oil.

Seafood
Shrimp, scallops, lobster, crab, clams, oysters. Use lemon juice, fat-free butter substitutes or cocktail sauce.

Eggs
Eggs (1 Egg Yolk and 4 Egg Whites), EggBeaters (4 ounces). Boil, poach, scramble or fry in PAM.

SALAD
When you are in ketosis, you are burning your own body fat. At this point, you may add two cups of salad, one or two times a day, with low-fat, low-carbohydrate dressing. Use only lettuce, cucumbers, onions, mushrooms, radishes and sprouts. No other vegetables. No carrots. No tomatoes. No corn. No potatoes. You need to stay in ketosis to lose weight!

CHEESE
After you are in ketosis, you may add cheese to your protein list. You may have up to two slices of low-fat cheese OR 3/4 cup

fat-free cottage cheese, up to three times a day. Remember: If you have three servings of cheese, you can't eat anything else from the protein list.

DIRECTIONS
Drink 128 ounces of water every day. This includes all the coffee, tea (no cream or creamer), club soda, diet soda and Diet Jello you want.

No diet Popsicles, no sugarless gum, no breath mints and no alcohol. Use Equal and Sweet 'N Low tablets only, no packets.

If cheese or salad knock you out of ketosis, return to the original protein-only diet (no cheese, no salad). Drink your water. You should be back in ketosis in two to three days. Then try only one serving of cheese or salad per day.

Cooking: Steam, boil, broil, bake or pan fry. Trim fat and remove skin before cooking. If the pan gets too dry, add a little broth or water. Season with salt, pepper, herbs, spices, cocktail sauce, fat-free mayonnaise, ketchup and mustard. If you are on a sodium-reduced diet, take it easy on the salt. Use low-fat and low-carbohydrate dressings. No breading.

If you crave sweets or starches, and diet soda and Diet Jello do not satisfy you, stop all diet soda, Diet Jello, poultry, eggs and cottage cheese for a few days. Your cravings should disappear.

Check your urine for ketosis at least 3 times a day. Use Ketostix. You should be in small or moderate ketosis. If you are in large ketosis, you are dehydrated and need to drink more non-caloric fluid immediately and then every day.

Exercise. Try to exercise at least 10 minutes every day. 45 minutes is better. You must break a sweat. Try three miles on a flat treadmill, at 3-6 mph, every day.

Option 2: Dr. Nagler's Ketogenic Crash

The second alternative to my 10-Days-10-Pounds-Off Program or my 500 Diet is actually the fastest diet of all, but difficult to stay on. Most of my patients lose five to 10 pounds their first week and in excess of five pounds every week on this program. This is the most radical of my crash diet programs.

Make sure that you drink at least 40 ounces of water with each meal. Each meal refers to every time you eat. You need to drink a minimum of at least 128 ounces of water every day, no matter what. **You may have up to two pounds of protein each day on this program.** Remember, you can have up to two pounds of meat each day. That's it. And if you're not hungry, don't eat. Here's the list.

MEAT
Up to two pounds each day of the following:

● Chicken
● Turkey
● Tuna

- Shrimp
- Crab
- Lobster
- Eggs (4 oz. EggBeaters or one whole egg with 3 egg whites)

The above can be fresh or canned and either broiled, baked or grilled. Poultry shouldn't have skin. Make a protein salad with a tablespoon of Miracle Whip Free. Add lemon juice when preparing the seafood salads.

When preparing the egg protein, use PAM. Serve scrambled, fried, as an omelet or make egg salad with a tablespoon of Miracle Whip Free.

You can lose five to 10 pounds a week on this diet. If you're not hungry, don't eat. Eat ONLY the foods on the list. NO cheating. Don't eat breakfast or anything at all until you are hungry.

DIRECTIONS
You must drink at least 12 large glasses of water (128 ounces) every day. Have all the coffee, tea (no cream or creamer), club

soda, diet soda and Diet Jello you want. This is a very, very rapid weight-loss program. Make sure you drink all of your water — at least 128 ounces a day; 150-200 ounces is better to help you feel your best. The water helps to block your appetite and wash out the fat you are burning. Avoid dehydration. You literally pee away your fat, so drink your water!

No diet Popsicles, sugarless gum, breath mints or alcohol. Equal and Sweet 'N Low tablets only, no packets.

Cooking: Steam, boil, broil, grill, bake or pan fry. Trim fat and remove skin before cooking. You can use up to one teaspoon of butter, margarine or oil if you're going nuts, but try to control yourself. Sprays like PAM are better. Using nonstick cookware makes it easier to cook with less fat. Season with salt, pepper, herbs, spices, lemon juice, cocktail sauce, fat-free mayonnaise, ketchup and mustard. If you are on a sodium-reduced diet, take it easy on the salt. Use low-fat, low-carbohydrate dressings. No breading.

If you crave sweets or starches, and diet soda and Diet Jello don't satisfy you, STOP ALL diet soda, Diet Jello, as well as all poultry and eggs for a few days. Believe it or not, your cravings should disappear.

Check your urine for ketosis three times a day. Use Ketostix to make sure you are in ketosis. You should be in small or moderate ketosis. If you are in large ketosis, you are dehydrated and need to drink more water immediately!

Option 3: Dr. Nagler's Rotation Diet

The last alternative to my 10-Days-10-Pounds-Off Program and Dr. Nagler's 500 Diet is my Rotation Diet. This program of rotating crash diets offers the most variety and also provides quick results. If you get easily bored on diets, Dr. Nagler's Rotation may be good for you.

There are two groups of crashes on the Rotation. The first group of crashes (Group I) are faster, because they are ketogenic, but they are a bit harder to stay on. You can switch back and forth between the Group I and Group II diets, but if you stick to the Rotations from Group I, you'll lose weight a little faster. Don't go on any of my Rotations without your personal physician's approval, supervision and monitoring.

To begin, select one of the rotation diets and stick to it for three days. Then switch to another diet on the list. After three days, switch again. Most of my patients lose at least five pounds a week on this program.

As with my other diet plans, you must drink at least 128 ounces of water a day on all of the Rotations. You may also have one cup of salad with fat-free dressing, two times a day if you're hungry. If you don't need the salad, please don't eat it. The salad will slow down your weight loss a bit, but usually not significantly. You may have ketchup and mustard (1 tablespoon of each per serving), and salt, pepper, herbs, spices and soy sauce. If you are on a sodium-reduced diet, take it easy one the salt and soy sauce.

Group I Rotations

The Group I Rotation diets are ketogenic and very, very fast. You should drop about a pound a day on them your first week, and at least five pounds every week.

Chicken Crash
You may have up to a whole chicken a day, or 13 ounces of canned chicken in broth. No skin. If you want to make chicken salad, you can use 1 tablespoon of Miracle Whip Free with a teaspoon of relish for every 6 ounces of chicken.

Tuna Torture
You may have up to 13 ounces of canned

tuna (packed in water, not oil) a day. To make tuna salad, you can use 1 tablespoon of Miracle Whip Free with 1 teaspoon of relish for every 6 ounces of tuna.

Shrimp Craze
Up to 2 pounds of shrimp, lobster or crab a day, with lemon and cocktail sauce. Add lettuce and make a salad. You may have up to 4 tablespoons of low-fat, low-carbohydrate dressing per day.

Hot Dog Diet
Up to 12 kosher 97 percent fat-free hot dogs a day, with mustard and ketchup.

Egg Crate
Up to six hard-boiled eggs a day. Salt, ketchup and mustard. If you are on a sodium-reduced diet, take it easy on the salt.

Grapefruit, Bacos and Eggs
Up to three grapefruit and up to three 4-ounce cartons of EggBeaters per day. You can add 1 tablespoon of Bacos to each serving of EggBeaters if you like. Cook with PAM.

Cheese Crash

Up to 1 pound of fat-free string, shredded or cottage cheese a day, with ketchup or mustard if you like.

Mickey Dee's Diet

Up to three McDonald's grilled chicken salads a day. NO croutons and NO dressing. Unlimited diet soda.

Arby's Diet

Up to 2 Big Montanas a day, no bun. 1 packet of ketchup or 1 packet Arby's Sauce per serving. All the Diet Coke you can drink.

Burger King Craze

Up to 3 meat-only Whoppers a day. No bun, no vegetables, no mayonnaise. One packet ketchup and one packet mustard per meat patty. Unlimited diet soda.

Group II Rotations

The Group II Rotations are very low fat and extremely fast, but not quite as fast as the Group I Rotations.

Yogurt Yelp

Up to six cups of fat-free, 100-calories-per-serving yogurt a day. Most people do best having 1-3 cups, whenever they are hungry. But no more than six cups per day.

Milk and Banana Blast

One banana with 8 ounces skim milk, blended together or not, up to four times a day.

Cereal Crash

Up to six 3/4-ounce boxes of pre-packaged cereal. You are allowed one 3/4 cup of skim milk per serving.

Cottage Cheese Crash

3/4 cup of fat-free cottage cheese, one fruit, two saltines — up to three times a day.

Strawberries and Cream Crash

One cup of strawberries with 1 tablespoon of fat-free yogurt or 1 tablespoon of diet Cool Whip Free, up to three times a day.

Baked Potato Blast

One baked potato, up to six times a day. Top your baked potatoes with ketchup or 1 tablespoon of non-fat yogurt or 1 tablespoon of non-fat sour cream. If you want to be exceedingly efficient, make your potatoes once a day in the morning in your microwave, or get them at Wendy's.

Rice Diet

This is one of my most popular Rotations. You can have two meals a day, lunch and dinner.

Lunch — 1 cup brown or white rice with 1 cup fresh fruit (any kind of fruit, as long as it's fresh). Some people like to chop their fruit and mix it into the rice.

Dinner — 1 cup brown or white rice with 1 cup steamed vegetable (any type of vegetable you want). Some people like to chop their vegetable and mix it into the rice.

Season with salt or soy sauce. However, if you are on a sodium-reduced diet, use a light hand with both. To make it easy for yourself, cook three days' worth of rice in advance (2 cups of cooked rice a day) in a rice cooker, in the microwave or on the stove.

I recommend using brown rice over white (or a 50-50 combination). Brown rice has a lot of fiber and is very nutritious.

Section 3:

The Secret To Keeping Weight Off

Now That You've Lost Your Weight

Most people gain their weight back. From my experience this is true. But it doesn't have to be. There is a way to keep your weight off. It's simple. There are two cardinal rules that you must follow if you want to get down to your ideal weight and stay there:

(1) Stop eating the average American diet.

(2) Exercise 20-45 minutes a day three times a week.

You can't go back to eating the way you used to eat when you were overweight. If you do that, you'll gain back all of your weight in no time. To keep your weight off, you have to eat less than you ate before. That does not mean that you can never have a cookie or a piece of cake or even a slice of pizza. It's just that you can't have these treats very often or in large amounts.

You Can't Go Back To Your Old Ways

You have to stop eating garbage. Try to get off the average American diet. It's way too high in fat and calories. We could learn a lot from the Japanese. The Japanese have the longest life expectancy on the planet. This is due to Western medical care and an Oriental ultra low-fat diet of rice, fish, vegetables and seaweed. They hardly ever eat bread, butter, cheese, dairy products or dessert.

Unfortunately, the Japanese diet is hard to follow. Most Americans can't imagine giving up dairy products and bread. Plus, the thought of seaweed is unappealing to many people. If you eat out a lot, as most Americans do (three to four times a week), controlling your fat intake can also be a problem. Most restaurants cook with way too much butter and oil. Next time you go to a restaurant, sit at a table with a clear view of the kitchen. Watch how much oil, butter and sauce is used. Food generally glistens with fat. Portions are way too large, too.

What can you do to stay thin? I'll tell you what I do. To maintain my weight, I sweat my brains out in the basement for 45 minutes a day, five days a week, on my Schwinn elliptical machine. I'm next to Gabrielle (my wife), who is sweating it out on the treadmill. Even worse, more often than not, I live on rice, fish, vegetables and seaweed, too.

My full maintenance program is spelled out in *The Diet Doctor's Wife's Cookbook* available by calling 1-800-511-9769 and from www.dietresults.com.

Exercise And Weight Control

In addition to watching what you eat, it helps to exercise on a regular basis. Most people find it hard to follow a regular exercise program. Although many people belong to health and fitness clubs, most Americans (approximately 60 percent of the population) get no exercise on a regular basis. The pattern is one of fits and starts. How many times have you started an exercise regimen and found that after three months you lost interest? Or you just didn't have time to get to the club or go for a run or whatever?

In my practice, the best predictor of whether a patient will start and stick to an exercise program is whether that person is already following an exercise program at the time he or she walks into my office. I recommend exercising for 20-45 minutes a day, three to five times per week and a combination of resistance and cardiovascular exercise. Whether you choose to use a treadmill, an elliptical machine or go to an aerobics class, try to break a sweat for at least 20 minutes a day three times a week.

Exercise helps to speed up your metabolism and change your setpoint (See page 29), so you can maintain your weight. Interval training is another way to exercise and get the most from a cardiovascular program. Interval training can cause your body to burn more calories after exercise than it normally does. To do interval training, warm up by walking on a treadmill at an easy pace for five minutes. For the next 20 minutes, alternate between running for 30 seconds and walking for 60 seconds. Cool down by walking for five minutes. Try this workout once a week.

The other exercise-based way to reset your setpoint is to build muscle. The more muscle you have, the more calories you burn at rest. Try to add weight training to your exercise program at least twice a week. You can read fitness magazines to get different workouts or use the one that follows.

No-Brainer Maintenance Resistance-Training Program

This program uses a resistance band, which can be purchased at most sporting goods stores.

Exercise	Sets	Reps
Squat	2	10-15
Chest Press	2	10-15
Back Row	2	10-15
Biceps Curl	2	10-15
Bench Dip	2	10-15
Crunch	2	10-15

Exercise Instructions

Squat

With one end of a resistance band in each hand, stand on the band with your knees slightly bent and your feet hip width apart. Pull the band so that the ends are at your shoulders. Squat down, pushing your hips back as if you were sitting in a chair. Bring your thighs parallel to the ground and make sure your knees don't go back to your toes. Squeeze your butt (or glutes, as those muscles are called) as you press back up. Repeat for as many repetitions as necessary.

Chest Press

Stand erect with your feet hip-width apart. Wrap the resistance band around your back, with one end in each hand. Your arms should be shoulder level and bent at a 90-degree angle. Press the resistance ends away from your body, then slowly return to the bent-arm position. Repeat for necessary reps.

Back Row

Sit erect on the floor with your legs stretched in front of you. Wrap the resistance band around your feet. Grasp one end of the band with each hand. Keep your knees slightly bent, your torso upright, your abs tight and your lower back slightly arched. Pull the band toward your lower abdomen, keeping your arms close to the sides of your body. Bring your shoulder blades together at the end of the movement. The rowing motion should come from your upper back, not your arms or lower back. Slowly allow your arms to extend and return the band to the starting position, without leaning forward at the finish. Repeat for necessary reps.

Shoulder Press

Stand in the middle of the resistance band and grasp each ends. Hold the band above your shoulders, behind your arms. Begin with your upper arms parallel to the floor. Press your arms overhead, stopping just short of locking. Slowly lower your arms back to the starting position. Repeat for necessary reps.

Biceps Curl

Stand in the middle of the resistance band and grasp each end with your hands. Hold the ends at your sides with a neutral grip, palms facing your thighs. Keep your elbows close to your sides. As you curl the band toward your shoulders, slowly turn your hands out so that your palms face the ceiling at the top position. Lower the band back to the starting position. Repeat for necessary reps.

Bench Dip

Position yourself with your hands on the edge of a bench, with your feet on the floor in front of you. Begin with your arms straight but not locked. With your body upright (not leaning forward), slowly lower yourself until your upper arms are parallel to the floor. Press back up to the starting position, squeezing your triceps at the top. Repeat for necessary reps.

Crunch

Lie on the floor with your knees bent and hands behind your head. Curl up, bringing your torso toward your knees, concentrating on crunching your abdominal muscles as you come up. Try to get your shoulder blades off the floor. Don't pull on your head or press your chin into your chest. Repeat for necessary reps.

Dr. Nagler's No-Brainer Maintenance Program

My No-Brainer Maintenance Program gives you a foundation diet for keeping weight off. It is the diet that you should follow most of the time. Some people follow it five days a week and cheat a little on the weekends. Some people follow it six days a week. Some people follow it every day except holidays, birthdays and vacation.

This program will help you keep your weight off longer. If you follow it religiously, you should have no trouble keeping off every ounce you have lost for good. The program is easy, so you won't feel like you are on maintenance. None of your friends will ever know unless you tell them.

The 15 No-Brainer Rules

1. **Drink as much non-caloric fluid as you can, at least 128 ounces a day.** Keep your fluid intake up. Never get dehydrated.

2. **When you think you are hungry, drink something first.** Before a meal or any time you eat have 20 ounces of non-caloric fluid. If your hunger goes away, don't eat. If you're still hungry after the 20 ounces, fill up on vegetables first.

3. **If you're not hungry, don't eat.**

4. **The less you eat, the easier it will be for you to keep your weight off.** Keep your portions small. Think about serving sizes. Protein shouldn't be much larger than a deck of cards. Stay away from bread and cheese like the plague.

5. **Take it easy on butter, margarine and oil.**

6. **Avoid fried foods and breading.**

7. **Stay away from beer, wine and alcohol.** These beverages stimulate appetite.

8. **Stay away from yeasted flour products.** It is almost impossible to keep your weight under control if you eat yeasted flour — bread, crackers, pizza or pasta.

Take it easy on cookies, cakes and pies. Baked yeasted flour raises your insulin level and makes you hungry.

9. **Instead of yeasted baked flour, have oatmeal, popcorn, brown rice or baked potatoes.** Whole foods keep you fuller longer. Use non-fat, low-fat, low-calorie toppings. Use ketchup, soy sauce and butter-flavored spray.

10. **Take it easy on fruit.** It's almost impossible to keep weight off eating more than two to three pieces of fruit a day. Your insulin level can go way up, which can make you hungry and crave sweets and starches.

11. **Avoid fruit juice.** An average glass of fruit juice is extracted from approximately four servings of fruit. That's enough fruit for two days.

12. **Get your protein mostly from fish.** Eat mostly salmon, tuna, swordfish, seafood, shrimp, lobster, crab, etc. Try to limit all protein (fish, beef, pork, poultry) to no more than a pound a day.

13. **If you don't like fish or shellfish, beware of chicken or turkey.** Poultry can trigger terrible sweet and starch cravings. Watch yourself.

14. **Have beef, pork or lamb no more than twice a week.** Avoid red meat entirely if you can, since it tends to be the fattiest of all protein. If you do decide to eat red meat, choose the leanest cuts such as filet mignon or tenderloin for beef, and tenderloin and loin chop for pork.

15. **Keep your intake of Equal, Sweet 'N Low, breath mints and sugarless gum to a minimum.** Artificial sweeteners can also trigger sweet and starch cravings and make you overeat.

So What About Cheating?

There will be times (given that you're human) that you will cheat. Don't let yourself get out of control. Don't cheat very often and, when you do, keep your portions small.

Not cheating very often means different things to different people. When you first start maintenance, be conservative. If you are going to cheat, cheat on one thing once a week. For example, have a glass of wine on the weekend. Experiment. Everyone is different.

A word of caution: Cheating on one thing can trigger your desire to cheat on something else. You can lose control and gain weight. To avoid this problem, follow my No-Brainer Maintenance Program exactly as written and listen to your Motivating Implosion tape (See page 171) every day.

MENU SUGGESTIONS

BREAKFAST
1 cup of oatmeal, sliced bananas,
coffee or tea

or

6 egg whites or 4 oz. EggBeaters omelet,
coffee or tea

or

1 cup Bran Flakes, 1/2 cup non-fat milk,
coffee or tea

or

Piece of fruit, coffee or tea

LUNCH

4 oz. tuna with 1 Tbsp. fat-free
mayonnaise, rice cake, 1 medium apple,
coffee or tea

or

Shrimp cocktail: six jumbo shrimp and
1/2 cup of cocktail sauce,
1/2 cantaloupe, coffee or tea

or

1 cup steamed vegetables, 1 cup brown
rice, coffee or tea

or

Omelet: six egg whites or 4 oz.
EggBeaters, 1 oz. fat-free cheese and
vegetables, 1 cup salad with 1 Tbsp. low-
fat dressing, berries, coffee or tea

DINNER
6 oz. broiled fish, 1 cup steamed
vegetables, 1 medium baked potato,
coffee or tea

or

1 cup vegetable soup, 4 oz. roast turkey,
1 cup salad with 1 Tbsp. low-fat
dressing, berries, coffee or tea

or

6 oz baked chicken, 1 cup steamed
vegetables, 1 medium baked apple,
coffee or tea

or

6 grilled shrimp, 1 cup grilled vegetables,
1/2 cup brown or white rice, 1 cup
salad with 1 Tbsp. low-fat dressing,
coffee or tea

Section 4

Section A

Diet Results

Products that help block your appetite, speed up fat-burning and triple your weight loss with exercise.

If you want to lose weight even faster on my 10-Days-10-Pounds-Off Program or Dr. Nagler's 500 Diet, you can do the same thing my patients do at my office — take Diet Results Packs, Fat Packs and Exercise Packs.

Diet Results Packs

When a patient tells me that they want to lose weight even faster, the first thing I do is have them take a Diet Results Pack three times a day.

Diet Results Packs are my specially for-mulated combination of appetite suppres-sants and fat burners designed to make you less hungry, speed fat burning and boost your energy while you are dieting. You take two pills in the morning, two pills at noon and two pills at 6 p.m. My patients lose weight faster and feel better when they add a Diet Result Pack to my programs.

Diet Results Packs are available by calling 734-422-8040 in Detroit and 800-511-9769 and from www.dietresults.com.

Fat Packs

The second thing you can do to speed up your weight loss is to add Fat Packs. Fat Packs are my specially formulated combinations of amino acids and supplements designed to speed up fat burning and move the scale faster. Fat Packs help you lose weight faster by enzymatically facilitating the breakdown of body fat. A nice side effect is that they can also help curb your sweet and starch cravings. You can take a Fat Pack once, twice (or if you are in a real hurry) three times a day to move the scale faster.

Fat Packs are available by calling 734-422-8040 in Detroit and 800-511-9769 and from www.dietresults.com.

Exercise Packs

If someone asks me, "What's the single best thing I can do to really speed up my weight loss?" I always say: Exercise Packs. Exercise Packs are my special amino acid complex capsules, designed to triple fat-burning and inch loss with exercise.

The good news is that my Exercise Packs are my fastest way to burn more inches and really move the scale. The bad news is that Exercise Packs absolutely do not work unless you are exercising.

Here's how to use Exercise Packs to really speed your weight loss:

Make sure that you are exercising hard enough to break a sweat, at least 20 minutes a day. Forty-five minutes of exercise is even better, but 20 minutes will do it.

About an hour before you exercise, take one Exercise Pack. In addition, take another Exercise Pack at bedtime. If you only want to take an Exercise Pack once, take the bedtime dose. It's the most important. If you forget to take the Exercise Pack an hour before you exercise, take it right before you exercise. If you totally forget to take the Exercise Pack before you exercise, you can even take it right after. Exercise-Packs are the single best thing you can do to accelerate your weight loss, but don't take them unless you are exercising. Taking Exercise Packs won't hurt you if you are not exercising, they just don't help you lose weight.

Exercise Packs are available by calling 734-422-8040 in Detroit and 800-511-9769 and from www.dietresults.com.

Diet Packs

Diet Packs are my special prepackaged packets of tablets and capsules, designed to help specific diet problems. For example, some Diet Packs help stop bingeing. Other Diet Packs help kill sweet cravings. Other Diet Packs help curb starch cravings. Others help boost your energy. Most patients take Diet Packs once, twice or three times a day, depending on individual need.

Here is a complete list of all Diet Packs available. You can use Diet Packs to help solve specific problems, feel better and accelerate your weight loss on all of my programs.

- **Binge-Pack** — stop night eating and binging, stabilize blood sugar
- **Cold-Pack** — fight off colds and the flu in just a few days
- **Depression-Pack** — lift depression, improve mood, calm anxiety
- **Diet Results Pack** — block your appetite, speed up fat burning
- **Dry-Pack** — help dry hair, improve dry skin, revitalize your nails

- **Energy-Pack** — boost energy and increase vitality without jitters
- **Exercise-Pack** — increase fat burning and inch loss with exercise
- **Fat-Pack** — increase fat burning, curb cravings, move the scale
- **Hair-Pack** — put luster and shine back, eliminate brittleness
- **Hormone-Pack** — eliminate hot flashes, night sweats, PMS symptoms
- **Red-White-Blue** — amino acids to curb cravings & speed fat burning
- **Sex-Pack** — get your sex drive back, boost your sexual cravings
- **Sleep-Pack** — stop insomnia, sleep disturbances and night eating
- **Starch-Pack** — eliminate bread, cracker, chip and starch cravings
- **Sweet-Pack** — block cravings for candy, ice cream and cake
- **Vitamin-Pack** — boost your immune system with anti-oxidants

Diet Packs are available by calling 734-422-8040 in Detroit and 800-511-9769 and from www.dietresults.com.

The Super Crash Diet

Dr. Nagler's Formula

Dr. Nagler's Formula is my activated amino acid complex drink, designed to really speed up fat-burning, boost your energy and make you feel full. Formula is absolutely the fastest way I know to lose weight.

Most people lose more than a pound a day, more than five to 10 pounds their first week on Formula. Weight drops off as fast as medically possible, without hunger or cravings or drop in energy. Formula is my most popular program. It's the easiest diet I have and most of my patients feel absolutely terrific on it.

Formula comes in a single-serving size carton with a straw, like a juice box. It's ready to drink and requires no refrigeration. There are three flavors: vanilla, chocolate and strawberry.

My Formula Program is easy to follow: You drink two Formula, twice a day. Most people drink two Formula for lunch and two Formula for dinner. But it doesn't matter when you drink your Formula. You will feel better and you will do better on the program if you force yourself to four servings of Formula a day, whether you feel you need it or want it or not.

If you are hungry you may have an additional two Formula a day for breakfast and/or an evening snack. Most people do better having two formula at a time, not one. No more than eight Formula per day. Four Formula a day is best; six Formula a day is OK; eight Formula, you're pushing it.

You must drink at least 128 ounces (one gallon) of non-caloric fluid a day on this program, in addition to your Formula. You need this much fluid to flush out the fat you are burning, and to keep your kidneys healthy.

Drink water, diet soda, coffee or tea — as much as you can and as much as you want. Make sure you drink a minimum of 128 ounces of fluid a day, in addition to your Formula. No juice, milk, regular soda or creamer in your coffee or tea.

Absolutely no alcohol. It will stop you from losing weight.

No lozenges, cough drops, candy, or breath mints.

Use Breath Asure or Binaca spray for your breath.

Use Sweet 'N Low or Equal tablets only (no powdered packets).

Sugarless gum is OK, up to 12 sticks a day.

Doctor Nagler's Formula is available by calling 734-422-8040 in Detroit and 800-511-9769 and from www.dietresults.com.

My Best Crash Diet

Come and see me in Detroit.
Or visit the Diet Results near you.
Call 734-422-8040 in Detroit or 800-511-9769 or go to www.dietresults.com to find the Diet Results near you.

Dr. Nagler's Injection Program

Dr. Nagler's Injection Program is my flagship weight-loss program. It's the program I've used to help more than 12,000 patients lose weight over the past 20 years. It's my fastest, safest and best medically monitored weight-loss program.

How does Doctor Nagler's Injection Program work?

My program works by using strong, safe, prescription appetite suppressants to block your appetite and speed up fat-burning.

I use special Fat-Burning Injections designed to help speed up your weight loss.

I use special Craving Injections designed to help eliminate your sweet and starch cravings.

Finally, I use special Energy-Boosting Injections designed to help increase your vitality.

Dr. Nagler's Injection Program helps your body burn fat more efficiently, curbs your carbohydrate cravings and boosts your energy.

The cost of Dr. Nagler's Injection Program is $199.95 for your enrollment, and then just $65 a week. I think it's a bargain. For just $65, every week you get strong, safe prescription appetite suppressant medication and come to the office six days a week for your special Injections. Most patients melt.

How often do I have to come to your office?

You come to my Detroit office every day, six days a week — Monday through Saturday, for your Injections. If you can't make it to the office every day, come every other day. The fastest weight loss occurs with daily Injections. But you can still lose weight very rapidly and feel terrific on the program by receiving your Injections every other day.

How much weight should I lose?

You should lose about half a pound per Injection. Most patients lose five to 10 pounds their first week on the program, and about five pounds every week thereafter. My record weight loss is 40 pounds in one week for a man and 26 pounds in one week for a woman. You probably won't lose this much, but it is not uncommon for many patients to lose 10-15 pounds their first week on the Super-Saver Injection Program.

What's in the Injections?

Lipotropic Agents, Energy Boosters and Craving Modulators.

Lipotropic agents are a class of substances that play important roles in the body's use and breakdown of fat. Many substances have lipotropic properties. Through their involvement in lipid (fat) metabolism, lipotropics help maintain a healthy liver. I use a combination of amino acids, minerals, vitamins and medication in my injections to help boost energy, control sweet and starch cravings and facilitate fat-burning.

Call 734-422-8040 in Detroit or 800-511-9769 or go to www.dietresults.com to find the Diet Results near you.

Implosion Tapes

My Implosion Tapes will help you stay on my 500 Diet and 10-Days-10-Pounds-Off Program without cheating. The tapes provide the psychological motivation to keep you dieting and kill your cravings.

All of my Implosion Tapes are available directly from my office to help you stay on my 10-Days-10-Pounds-Off-Program or 500 Diet.

The tapes contain implosion imagery to make you lose your cravings for sweets and starches, and to keep you motivated, focused and energetic while dieting.

There is a single tape Motivating Implosion for Weight Loss:

1 — Motivating Implosion for Weight Loss

There are five six-tape Implosion sets available for Weight Loss:

2 — Motivating Implosion to Keep You On Your Diet

3 — Positive Implosion for Sweets

4 — Positive Implosion for Starches

5 — Negative Implosion for Sweets

6 — Negative Implosion for Starches

All tapes are recorded continuously, so you should only have to rewind once a week.

There are two six-tape Implosion sets for Smoking and Drinking:

7 — Implosion to Quit Smoking

8 — Implosion to Stop Drinking

Implosion Tapes are available by calling 734-422-8040 in Detroit and 800-511-9769 and from www.dietresults.com.

Books by Bill Nagler, M.D.

Doctor Nagler's Crash Diet

Doctor Nagler's Super-Saver Injection Program

The Diet Doctor's Wife's Cookbook (with Gabrielle Nagler)

The Lindner Manuals for Weight Loss

The Dirty Half Dozen

Audio Tapes, CDs and Computer Programs

Hypnosis for Weight Loss

Hypnosis to Stop Smoking

Hypnosis to Stop Drinking

Motivating Implosion 6-Tape Set

Motivating Implosion Single Tape

Positive Implosion for Sweets

Positive Implosion for Starches

Negative Implosion for Sweets

Negative Implosion for Starches

Living Well is the Best Medicine

Brainwashing Weight Reduction Seminar

Brainwashing Graduate Reinforcement Tape

Books, tapes, CDs and other products are all available by calling 734-422-8040 in Detroit and 800-511-9769 and from www.dietresults.com.

Appendix 1:

Dr. Nagler's Crash Diet Tear-out Sheets

Dr. Nagler's 10-Days-10-Pounds-Off-Program Summary

BREAKFAST
1/2 Grapefruit
Coffee or Tea

LUNCH
1/2 Grapefruit
Salad (2 cups)
Omelet made with EggBeaters OR 4 Egg
Whites, 1 Egg Yolk and Bacos

DINNER
1/2 Grapefruit
Salad (2 cups)
Vegetable (1 cup)
Meat (8 ounces)

Salad with 2 Tbsp. low-fat, low-carbohydrate dressing:
● Lettuce (Darker greens like romaine and mesclun have more nutrients and fiber.)

- Cucumbers
- Mushrooms
- Onions
- Radishes
- Sprouts

Vegetables

- Asparagus
- Broccoli
- Brussels sprouts
- Cauliflower
- Mushrooms
- Sauerkraut
- Spinach
- String beans

Meat

- Chicken
- Clams
- Crab
- Fish (any type)
- Lobster
- Mussels
- Sardines
- Scallops
- Shrimp
- Turkey
- Veal
- Water-packed tuna

1 — Get your doctor's approval first.

2 — No alcohol or coffee creamer.

3 — Drink about 128 ounces of water or other no-calorie beverage each day.

4 — No breading, butter, margarine or oil.

5 — Don't eat anything else.

Dr. Nagler's 10-Days-10-Pounds-Off-Program Summary

BREAKFAST
1/2 Grapefruit
Coffee or tea

LUNCH
1/2 Grapefruit
Salad (2 cups)
Omelet made with EggBeaters OR 4 Egg
Whites, 1 Egg Yolk and Bacos

DINNER
1/2 Grapefruit
Salad (2 cups)
Vegetable (1 cup)
Meat (8 ounces)

Salad with 2 Tbsp. low-fat, low-carbohy-drate dressing:
● Lettuce (Darker greens like romaine and mesclun have more nutrients and fiber.)

- Cucumbers
- Mushrooms
- Onions
- Radishes
- Sprouts

Vegetables
- Asparagus
- Broccoli
- Brussels sprouts
- Cauliflower
- Mushrooms
- Sauerkraut
- Spinach
- String beans

Meat
- Chicken
- Clams
- Crab
- Fish (any type)
- Lobster
- Mussels
- Sardines
- Scallops
- Shrimp
- Turkey
- Veal
- Water-packed tuna

1 — Get your doctor's approval first.

2 — No alcohol or coffee creamer.

3 — Drink about 128 ounces of water or other no-calorie beverage each day.

4 — No breading, butter, margarine or oil.

5 — Don't eat anything else.

Dr. Nagler's 500 Diet Summary

Eat one meal twice a day.

Each meal consists of a meat, a vegetable and a fruit.

If you prefer fresh food and want to cook, weigh everything before you eat it.

Canned meats and vegetables are faster and easier.

Meat: One 4-6 ounce serving of:
chicken, clams, crab, lobster, mussels, sardines, shrimp, tuna or turkey.

Vegetable: One 8 ounce water-packed can or 1 cup of:
asparagus, broccoli, brussels sprouts, cauliflower, mushrooms, sauerkraut, spinach or string beans.

Fruit: Fresh only (not canned):
1 apple, 1/2 cantaloupe, 12 grapes, 1/2 grapefruit, 1 orange or 6 strawberries.

1 — Get your doctor's approval first.
2 — No alcohol or creamers.
3 — No lozenges, gum or mints.
4 — Only Breath Asure or Binaca spray.
5 — Sweet 'N Low/Equal tablets only.
6 — Drink 4 quarts (128 ounces) water.
7 — Don't eat anything else.

Dr. Nagler's 500 Diet
Summary

Eat one meal twice a day.

Each meal consists of a meat, a vegetable and a fruit.

If you prefer fresh food and want to cook, weigh everything before you eat it.

Canned meats and vegetables are faster and easier.

Meat: One 4-6 ounce serving of:
chicken, clams, crab, lobster, mussels, sardines, shrimp, tuna or turkey.

Vegetable: One 8 ounce water-packed can or 1 cup of:
asparagus, broccoli, brussels sprouts, cauliflower, mushrooms, sauerkraut, spinach or string beans.

Fruit: Fresh only (not canned):
1 apple, 1/2 cantaloupe, 12 grapes, 1/2 grapefruit, 1 orange or 6 strawberries.

1 — Get your doctor's approval first.
2 — No alcohol or creamers.
3 — No lozenges, gum or mints.
4 — Only Breath Asure or Binaca spray.
5 — Sweet 'N Low/Equal tablets only.
6 — Drink 4 quarts (128 ounces) water.
7 — Don't eat anything else.

Appendix 2:

Implosion Therapy Scripts

Motivating Implosion Script

Close your eyes. Now. In your mind's eye. See yourself thin. (5 second pause.) Really see yourself thin. (5 second pause.) See yourself looking exactly the way you want to look. (5 second pause.) See yourself wearing exactly what you want to wear. (5 second pause.) See yourself in the mirror, strong and slender, and exactly the way you want to be. (5 second pause.) See yourself hungry, relaxed, not eating and in control. (5 second pause.)

Now. Feel yourself thin. (5 second pause.) Feel slim. (5 second pause.) Feel what it feels like to wear exactly what you want to wear. (5 second pause). Feel what it feels like to be thin and powerful and in control. (5 second pause.) Feel exactly the way you want to feel. (5 second pause.) Feel strong and slender, feel exactly the way you want to feel. (5 second pause.) Feel yourself hungry, not eating and in control. (5 second pause.)

Now. Be thin. (5 second pause.) Really, be slim. (5 second pause.) Be exactly what you want to be. (5 second pause.) Be strong and slender, and in control. (5 second pause.) Be thin, and hungry, not eating and in control. (5 second pause.) Be thin, and hungry, not eating and in control. (5 second pause.) Be thin, and hungry, not eating and in control. (5 second pause.) Now, open your eyes.

Positive Implosion Script 1 - Cake

Close your eyes. Now. See your favorite cake in front of you. (5 second pause.) Really see it. (5 second pause.) Look at it. (5 second pause.) Smell it. (5 second pause.) Now, take a knife and cut yourself a slice. (5 second pause.) Put the slice on a plate in front of you. (5 second pause.) See it. (5 second pause.) Really see it. (5 second pause.) Smell it. (5 second pause.) Now, take a fork and pick up a perfect mouthful. (5 second pause.) Look at it. (5 second pause.) Really see it. (5 second pause.)

Now, take a bite and slowly savor it. (5 second pause). Chew and swallow. (5 second pause.) Take another bite. (5 second pause.) Enjoy it. (5 second pause.) Take another. (5 second pause.) Enjoy it. (5 second pause.) Feel completely satisfied. (5 second pause.) Feel totally satisfied. (5 second pause.) Feel completely in control. (5 second pause.) Now, open your eyes.

Positive Implosion Script 2 – Cookies

Close your eyes. Now. See your favorite cookie in front of you. (5 second pause.) Really see it. (5 second pause.) Look at it. (5 second pause.) Smell it. (5 second pause.) Now, break off a piece. (5 second pause.) Look at the piece in your hand. (5 second pause.) See it. (5 second pause.) Really see it. (5 second pause.) Smell it. (5 second pause.)

Now, put it in your mouth. (5 second pause.) Savor it, enjoy it. (5 second pause.) Take another bite. (5 second pause.) Love it. (5 second pause.) Take another bite. (5 second pause.) Enjoy it. (5 second pause.) Feel completely satisfied. (5 second pause.) Feel totally satisfied. (5 second pause.) Feel completely in control. (5 second pause.) Now, open your eyes.

Positive Implosion Script 3 – Pie

Close your eyes. Now. See your favorite pie in front of you. (5 second pause.) Really see it. (5 second pause.) Look at it. (5 second pause.) Smell it. (5 second pause.) Now, take a knife and cut yourself a slice. (5 second pause.) Put the slice on a plate in front of you. (5 second pause.) See it. (5 second pause.) Really see it. (5 second pause.) Smell it. (5 second pause.) Now, take a fork and cut yourself a perfect mouthful. (5 second pause.) Look at it. (5 second pause.) Really see it. (5 second pause.)

Now, take a bite and slowly savor it. (5 second pause.) Eat it, swallow. (5 second pause.) Take another bite. (5 second pause.) Enjoy it. (5 second pause.) Take another. (5 second pause.) Enjoy it. (5 second pause.) Feel completely satisfied. (5 second pause.) Feel totally satisfied. (5 second pause.) Feel completely in control. (5 second pause.) Now, open your eyes.

Positive Implosion Script 4 – Ice Cream

Close your eyes. Now. See your favorite ice cream in a dish in front of you. (5 second pause.) Really see it. (5 second pause.) Look at it. (5 second pause.) Smell it. (5 second pause.) Now, take a spoonful. (5 second pause.) See it. (5 second pause.) Really see it. (5 second pause.) Smell it. (5 second pause.) Look at it. (5 second pause.)

Now, put the spoonful in your mouth. Savor it, eat it, enjoy it. (5 second pause.) Take another spoonful. (5 second pause.) Enjoy it. (5 second pause.) Take another spoonful. (5 second pause.) Enjoy it. (5 second pause.) Feel completely satisfied. (5 second pause.) Feel totally satisfied. (5 second pause.) Feel completely in control. (5 second pause.) Now, open your eyes.

Positive Implosion Script 5 – Candy

Close your eyes. Now. See your favorite candy in front of you. (5 second pause.) Really see it. (5 second pause.) Look at it. (5 second pause.) Smell it. (5 second pause.) Now, take a piece. (5 second pause.) Look at the piece in your hand. (5 second pause.) See it. (5 second pause.) Really see it. (5 second pause.) Smell it. (5 second pause.)

Now, put it in your mouth. (5 second pause.) Savor it, enjoy it. (5 second pause.) Take another piece. (5 second pause.) Love it. (5 second pause.) Take another piece. (5 second pause.) Enjoy it. (5 second pause.) Feel completely satisfied. (5 second pause.) Feel totally satisfied. (5 second pause.) Feel completely in control. (5 second pause.) Now, open your eyes.

Positive Implosion Script 6 – Pastry

Close your eyes. Now. See your favorite pastry in front of you. (5 second pause.) Really see it. (5 second pause.) Look at it. (5 second pause.) Smell it. (5 second pause.) Take a fork and cut off a piece. (5 second pause.) Look at the piece of pastry. (5 second pause.) See it. (5 second pause.) Really see it. (5 second pause.) Smell it. (5 second pause.)

Now, put it in your mouth. (5 second pause.) Savor it, enjoy it. (5 second pause.) Take another bite. (5 second pause.) Love it. (5 second pause.) Take another bite. (5 second pause.) Enjoy it. (5 second pause.) Feel completely satisfied. (5 second pause.) Feel totally satisfied. (5 second pause.) Feel completely in control. (5 second pause.) Now, open your eyes.

Positive Implosion Script 7 – Bread

Close your eyes. Now. See a loaf of your favorite bread in front of you. (5 second pause.) Really see it. (5 second pause.) Look at it. (5 second pause.) Smell it. (5 second pause.) Now, cut yourself a generous slice. (5 second pause.) Take the slice in your hand. Look at it. (5 second pause.) See it. (5 second pause.) Really see it. (5 second pause.) Smell it. (5 second pause.)

Now, take a bite. (5 second pause.) Savor it, enjoy it. (5 second pause.) Take another bite. (5 second pause.) Love it. (5 second pause.) Take another bite. (5 second pause.) Enjoy it. (5 second pause.) Feel completely satisfied. (5 second pause.) Feel totally satisfied. (5 second pause.) Feel completely in control. (5 second pause.) Now, open your eyes.

Positive Implosion Script 8 – Crackers

Close your eyes. Now. See your favorite type of cracker in front of you. (5 second pause.) Really see it. (5 second pause.) Look at it. (5 second pause.) Smell it. (5 second pause.) Now, break off a piece. (5 second pause.) Look at the piece of cracker in your hand. (5 second pause.) See it. (5 second pause.) Really see it. (5 second pause.) Smell it. (5 second pause.)

Now, put it in your mouth. (5 second pause.) Savor it, enjoy it. (5 second pause.) Take another bite. (5 second pause.) Love it. (5 second pause.) Enjoy it. (5 second pause.) Feel completely satisfied. (5 second pause.) Feel totally satisfied. (5 second pause.) Feel completely in control. (5 second pause.) Now, open your eyes.

Positive Implosion Script 9 – Chips

Close your eyes. Now. See a bowl of your favorite chips in front of you. (5 second pause.) Really see it. (5 second pause.) Look at it. (5 second pause.) Bring the bowl of chips up to your nose. Smell the chips. (5 second pause.) Now, take a chip. (5 second pause.) Look at the chip in your hand. (5 second pause.) See it. (5 second pause.) Really see it. (5 second pause.) Smell it. (5 second pause.)

Now, put it in your mouth. (5 second pause.) Savor it, enjoy it. (5 second pause.) Take another chip. (5 second pause.) Love it. (5 second pause.) Take another chip. (5 second pause.) Enjoy it. (5 second pause.) Feel completely satisfied. (5 second pause.) Feel totally satisfied. (5 second pause.) Feel completely in control. (5 second pause.) Now, open your eyes.

Positive Implosion Script 10 – Pizza

Close your eyes. Now. See your favorite pizza in front of you. (5 second pause.) Really see it. (5 second pause.) Look at it. (5 second pause.) Smell it. (5 second pause.) Pick up a slice. (5 second pause.) See the slice. (5 second pause.) Really see it. (5 second pause.) Smell it. (5 second pause.)

Now, take a bite. (5 second pause.) Savor it, enjoy it. (5 second pause.) Take another bite. (5 second pause.) Love it. (5 second pause.) Take another bite. (5 second pause.) Enjoy it. (5 second pause.) Feel completely satisfied. (5 second pause.) Feel totally satisfied. (5 second pause.) Feel completely in control. (5 second pause.) Now, open your eyes.

Positive Implosion Script 11 – Pasta

Close your eyes. Now. See a dish of your favorite pasta sitting in front of you. (5 second pause.) Really see it. (5 second pause.) Look at it. (5 second pause.) Smell it. (5 second pause.) Now, take a perfect forkful. (5 second pause.) See it. (5 second pause.) Really see it. (5 second pause.) Smell it. (5 second pause.)

Now, put it in your mouth, slowly savor it, eat it, swallow it. (5 second pause.) Take another forkful. (5 second pause.) Enjoy it. (5 second pause.) Take another. (5 second pause.) Enjoy it. (5 second pause.) Feel completely satisfied. (5 second pause.) Feel totally satisfied. (5 second pause.) Feel completely in control. (5 second pause.) Now, open your eyes.

Positive Implosion Script 12 – Potatoes

Close your eyes. Now. See your favorite potato dish in front of you. (5 second pause.) Really see it. (5 second pause.) Look at it. (5 second pause.) Smell it. (5 second pause.) Now, take a perfect forkful. (5 second pause.) See it. (5 second pause.) Really see it. (5 second pause.) Smell it. (5 second pause.)

Now, put it in your mouth, slowly savor it, eat it, swallow it. (5 second pause.) Take another bite. (5 second pause.) Enjoy it. (5 second pause.) Take another. (5 second pause.) Enjoy it. (5 second pause.) Feel completely satisfied. (5 second pause.) Feel totally satisfied. (5 second pause.) Feel completely in control. (5 second pause.) Now, open your eyes.

Negative Implosion Script 1 – Cake

Close your eyes. Now. See a slice of your favorite cake in front of you. (5 second pause.) Now, use a fork and cut a piece. Put it in your mouth and swallow it. (5 second pause.) As you go to take another bite, notice that there are worms coming out of the cake. (5 second pause.) There are worms coming out of your mouth. (5 second pause.) Look at the cake. There are worms coming out of the cake and out of your mouth. (5 second pause.) The worms are slimy and smell awful. (5 second pause.)

See yourself throw up. See yourself throw up worms and vomit all over the cake. (5 second pause.) Throw out the vomit-covered worm cake. Throw it out. (5 second pause.) It's gone. It's all gone. It's all gone. (5 second pause.) You don't need it anymore. (5 second pause.) You don't need it anymore. (5 second pause.) You don't need it anymore. (5 second pause.) Now, open your eyes.

Negative Implosion Script 2 – Cookies

Close your eyes. Now. See your favorite cookie in front of you. (5 second pause.) Now, put a piece in your mouth and swallow it. (5 second pause.) As you go to take another bite, notice that there are maggots coming out of the cookie. (5 second pause.) Maggots are coming out of your mouth. (5 second pause.) Look at the cookie. There are maggots coming out of the cookie and out of your mouth. (5 second pause.) The maggots are slimy and smell awful. (5 second pause.)

See yourself throw up. See yourself throw up maggots and vomit all over the cookie. (5 second pause.) Throw out the vomit-covered maggot cookie. Throw it out. (5 second pause.) It's gone. It's all gone. It's all gone. (5 second pause.) You don't need it anymore. (5 second pause.) You don't need it anymore. (5 second pause.) You don't need it anymore. (5 second pause.) Now, open your eyes.

Negative Implosion Script 3 – Pie

Close your eyes. Now. See a piece of your favorite pie in front of you. (5 second pause.) Now, use a fork and cut off a piece. Put it in your mouth and swallow it. (5 second pause.) As you go to take another bite, notice that there are worms coming out of the pie. (5 second pause.) Worms are coming out of your mouth. (5 second pause.) Look at the pie. There are worms coming out of the pie and out of your mouth. (5 second pause.) The worms are slimy and smell awful. (5 second pause.)

See yourself throw up. See yourself throw up worms and vomit all over the pie. (5 second pause.) Throw out the vomit-covered worm pie. Throw it out. (5 second pause.) It's gone. It's all gone. It's all gone. (5 second pause.) You don't need it anymore. (5 second pause.) You don't need it anymore. (5 second pause.) You don't need it anymore. (5 second pause.) Now, open your eyes.

Negative Implosion Script 4 – Ice Cream

Close your eyes. Now. See a dish of your favorite ice cream in front of you. (5 second pause.) Now, put a spoonful in your mouth and swallow it. (5 second pause.) As you take another spoonful, notice that there are worms coming out of the ice cream. (5 second pause.) Worms are coming out of your mouth. (5 second pause.) Look at the ice cream. There are worms coming out of the ice cream and out of your mouth. (5 second pause.) The worms are slimy and smell awful. (5 second pause.)

See yourself throw up. See yourself throw up worms and vomit all over the ice cream. (5 second pause.) Throw out the vomit-covered worm-infested ice cream. Throw it out. (5 second pause.) It's gone. It's all gone. It's all gone. (5 second pause.) You don't need it anymore. (5 second pause.) You don't need it anymore. (5 second pause.) You don't need it anymore. (5 second pause.) Now, open your eyes.

Negative Implosion Script 5 – Candy

Close your eyes. Now. See your favorite candy in front of you. (5 second pause.) Now, put a piece in your mouth and swallow it. (5 second pause.) As you go to take another bite, notice that there are maggots coming out of the candy. (5 second pause.) There are maggots coming out of your mouth. (5 second pause.) Look at the candy. There are maggots coming out of the candy and out of your mouth. (5 second pause.) The maggots are slimy and smell awful. (5 second pause.)

See yourself throw up. See yourself throw up maggots and vomit all over the candy. (5 second pause.) Throw out the vomit-covered maggot candy. Throw it out. (5 second pause.) It's gone. It's all gone. It's all gone. (5 second pause.) You don't need it anymore. (5 second pause.) You don't need it anymore. (5 second pause.) You don't need it anymore. (5 second pause.) Now, open your eyes.

Negative Implosion Script 6 – Pastry

Close your eyes. Now. See your favorite pastry in front of you. (5 second pause.) Now, put a piece in your mouth and swallow it. (5 second pause.) As you go to take another bite, notice that there are worms coming out of the pastry. (5 second pause.) There are worms coming out of your mouth. (5 second pause.) Look at the pastry. There are worms coming out of the pastry and out of your mouth. (5 second pause.) The worms are slimy and smell awful. (5 second pause.)

See yourself throw up. See yourself throw up worms and vomit all over the pastry. (5 second pause.) Throw out the vomit-covered worm pastry. Throw it out. (5 second pause.) It's gone. It's all gone. It's all gone. (5 second pause.) You don't need it anymore. (5 second pause.) You don't need it anymore. (5 second pause.) You don't need it anymore. (5 second pause.) Now, open your eyes.

Negative Implosion Script 7 – Bread

Close your eyes. Now. See a loaf of your favorite bread in front of you. (5 second pause.) Now, take a slice and put a piece in your mouth and swallow it. (5 second pause.) As you go to take another bite, notice that there are worms coming out of the bread. (5 second pause.) There are worms coming out of your mouth. (5 second pause.) Look at the bread. There are worms coming out of the bread and out of your mouth. (5 second pause.) The worms are slimy and smell awful. (5 second pause.)

See yourself throw up. See yourself throw up worms and vomit all over the bread. (5 second pause.) Throw out the vomit-covered worm bread. Throw it out. (5 second pause.) It's gone. It's all gone. It's all gone. (5 second pause.) You don't need it anymore. (5 second pause.) You don't need it anymore. (5 second pause.) You don't need it anymore. (5 second pause.) Now, open your eyes.

Negative Implosion Script 8 – Crackers

Close your eyes. Now. See a plate of your favorite crackers in front of you. (5 second pause.) Now, pick up one and take a bite. Chew and swallow. (5 second pause.) As you go to take another bite, notice that there are maggots coming out of the cracker. (5 second pause.) There are maggots coming out of your mouth. (5 second pause.) Look at the cracker. There are maggots coming out of the cracker and out of your mouth. (5 second pause.) The maggots are slimy and smell awful. (5 second pause.)

See yourself throw up. See yourself throw up maggots and vomit all over the cracker. (5 second pause.) Throw out the vomit-covered maggot cracker. Throw out all the crackers. (5 second pause.) They're gone. They're all gone. They're all gone. (5 second pause.) You don't need them anymore. (5 second pause.) You don't need them anymore. (5 second pause.) You don't need them anymore. (5 second pause.) Now, open your eyes.

Negative Implosion Script 9 – Chips

Close your eyes. Now. See a bowl of your favorite chips in front of you. (5 second pause.) Now, put a chip in your mouth, chew it and swallow it. (5 second pause.) As you go to take another one, notice that there are maggots coming out of the chips. (5 second pause.) There are maggots coming out of your mouth. (5 second pause.) Look at the chips. There are maggots coming out of the chips and out of your mouth. (5 second pause.) The maggots are slimy and smell awful. (5 second pause.)

See yourself throw up. See yourself throw up maggots and vomit all over the chips. (5 second pause.) Throw out the vomit-covered maggot chips. Throw them out. (5 second pause.) They're gone. They're all gone. They're all gone. (5 second pause.) You don't need them anymore. (5 second pause.) You don't need them anymore. (5 second pause.) You don't need them anymore. (5 second pause.) Now, open your eyes.

Negative Implosion Script 10 – Pizza

Close your eyes. Now. See your favorite type of pizza in front of you. (5 second pause.) Take a slice. (5 second pause.) Take a bite. Chew it and swallow it. (5 second pause.) As you go to take another bite, notice that there are worms coming out of the pizza. (5 second pause.) Worms are coming out of your mouth. (5 second pause.) Look at the pizza. There are worms coming out of the pizza and out of your mouth. (5 second pause.) The worms are slimy and smell awful. (5 second pause.)

See yourself throw up. See yourself throw up worms and vomit all over the pizza. (5 second pause.) Throw out the vomit-covered worm pizza. Throw it out. (5 second pause.) It's gone. It's all gone. It's all gone. (5 second pause.) You don't need it anymore. (5 second pause.) You don't need it anymore. (5 second pause.) You don't need it anymore. (5 second pause.) Now, open your eyes.

Negative Implosion Script 11 – Pasta

Close your eyes. Now. See your favorite pasta in front of you. (5 second pause.) Now, take a forkful. Put it in your mouth and swallow it. (5 second pause.) As you go to take another forkful, notice that there are worms coming out of the pasta. (5 second pause.) There are worms coming out of your mouth. (5 second pause.) Look at the pasta. There are worms coming out of the pasta and out of your mouth. (5 second pause.) The worms are slimy and smell awful. (5 second pause.)

See yourself throw up. See yourself throw up worms and vomit all over the pasta. (5 second pause.) Throw out the vomit-covered worm pasta. Throw it out. (5 second pause.) It's gone. It's all gone. It's all gone. (5 second pause.) You don't need it anymore. (5 second pause.) You don't need it anymore. (5 second pause.) You don't need it anymore. (5 second pause.) Now, open your eyes.

Negative Implosion Script 12 – Potatoes

Close your eyes. Now. See your favorite potato dish in front of you. (5 second pause.) Now, use a fork and take a bite. Chew and swallow. (5 second pause.) As you go to take another bite, notice that there are worms coming out of the potatoes. (5 second pause.) There are worms coming out of your mouth. (5 second pause.) Look at the potatoes. There are worms coming out of the potatoes and out of your mouth. (5 second pause.) The worms are slimy and smell awful. (5 second pause.)

See yourself throw up. See yourself throw up worms and vomit all over the potatoes. (5 second pause.) Throw out the vomit-covered worm potatoes. Throw it out. (5 second pause.) It's gone. It's all gone. It's all gone. (5 second pause.) You don't need it anymore. (5 second pause.) You don't need it anymore. (5 second pause.) You don't need it anymore. (5 second pause.) Now, open your eyes.

FOOTNOTES:

Section 1: The Virtue of Weight Cycling

1 http://www.niddk.nih.gov/health/nutrit/pubs/
health.htm; May 2, 2004. U.S. DEPARTMENT OF
HEALTH AND HUMAN SERVICES, National
Institutes of Health NIH Publication No. 03-4098,
November 2003.

2 Graci, S., Izzo, G, Savino, S., et al. Weight cycling
and cardiovascular risk factors in obesity.
International Journal of Obesity, 28: 65-71, 2004.

3 Lantz, H., Pelton, M., Liselotte, A., Torgerson, J.S. A
Dietary and behavioural programme for the treatment of obesity. A 4-year clinical trial and a long-
term posttreatment follow-up. *Journal of Internal
Medicine*, 254: 272-279, 2003.

4 Rowley, B. Winning the Weight Loss Game. *Muscle
& Fitness Hers*, 2(6): 66-69, 2002.

5 Nagler, W., Androff, A. Investigating the impact of
deconditioning anxiety on weight loss.
Psychological Reports, 66:595-600, 1990.

Section 2: Dr. Nagler's Crash Diets

6 Street, C. Internal Inferno: Help, hype or harm?
The fit female's guide to fat-burning supplements.
Muscle & Fitness Hers, 1(2): 63, 2000.

7 Elliot, T. Grapefruit: A great fruit for fat loss.
Muscle & Fitness, 65(5): 223, 2004.

INDEX

Order These Great Celebrity Books:

Please send the books checked below:

	Price Ea.	Qty.	Total
☐ *Freak!* – Inside the twisted mind of Michael Jackson	$5.99		
☐ *Divinely Decadent* – Liza Minnelli The drugs, the sex & the truth behind her bizarre marriage	$5.99		
☐ *Rosie O!* – How she conned America	$5.99		
☐ *J. Lo* – The secrets behind Jennifer Lopez's climb to the top	$5.99		
☐ *Pam* – The life and loves of Pamela Anderson	$5.99		
☐ *Julia Roberts* – America's sweetheart	$5.99		
☐ *The Richest Girl in the World* – Athina Onassis Roussel	$5.99		
☐ *Britney* – Not That Innocent	$5.99		
☐ *The Keanu Matrix* – Unraveling the puzzle of Hollywood's reluctant superstar	$5.99		
☐ *Demi* – The naked truth	$5.99		
☐ *Cruise Control* – The inside story of Hollywood's Top Gun	$5.99		
☐ *Johnny Cash* – An American legend	$5.99		
☐ *Sex, Drugs & Rock 'n' Roll* – The Lisa Marie Presley Story	$5.99		
Postage & Handling: U.S., $ 2.75 for one book, $ 1.00 for each additional			
Total enclosed:			

Ship to:

NAME _____

ADDRESS _____

CITY _____ STATE _____ ZIP _____

Please make your check or money order payable to AMI Books and mail it along with this order form to AMI Mail Order Books, 1000 American Media Way, Boca Raton, FL 33464-1000. Allow 4-6 weeks for delivery. Payable in U.S. funds only. No cash or COD accepted. We accept check or money orders ($15.00 fee for returned check). **Offer not available in Canada.**

0604IWL

About The Author

Bill Nagler, M.D., is Detroit's diet doctor. Dr. Nagler has specialized in weight control medicine for more than 20 years.

He is a graduate of the University of Michigan, the University of California and a Harvard Fellowship. He is a Diplomate of the American Board of Bariatric (Weight Control) Medicine and a Diplomate of the American Board of Psychiatry and Neurology.

Dr. Nagler has appeared on *The Phil Donahue Show*, *The Joan Rivers Show*, *The Sally Jessy Raphael*, *Larry King Live*, *CBS This Morning*, the *Montel Williams* show, the *Jenny Jones* show and *Jerry Springer*. He is the author of *Dr. Nagler's Crash Diet*, *Dr. Nagler's Super-Saver Injection Program* and co-author of *The Diet Doctor's Wife's Cookbook*. He has been featured in *USA Today*, *Cosmopolitan* and *Self* magazine.